John Merrylees, B. London

Carlsbad and its Environs

John Merrylees, B. London

Carlsbad and its Environs

ISBN/EAN: 9783337060534

Printed in Europe, USA, Canada, Australia, Japan

Cover: Foto ©ninafisch / pixelio.de

More available books at **www.hansebooks.com**

CARLSBAD

AND ITS ENVIRONS

BY

JOHN MERRYLEES

AUTHOR OF
"THE ENGLISHMAN'S GUIDE TO THE UNITED STATES AND CANADA,"
"PATERSON'S UNITED KINGDOM," "SWITZERLAND," ETC.

WITH

A Medical Treatise on the Use of the Waters

BY

B. LONDON, M.D.

RESIDENT PHYSICIAN AT CARLSBAD

With Fourteen Illustrations, and Plan of Carlsbad and Environs

LONDON
SAMPSON LOW, MARSTON, SEARLE, & RIVINGTON
CROWN BUILDINGS, 188 FLEET STREET, E.C.
1886

[All rights reserved]

Ballantyne Press
BALLANTYNE, HANSON AND CO.
EDINBURGH AND LONDON

PREFACE.

IN the preparation of this handbook it has been the aim of the Author to supply English-speaking visitors to Carlsbad with such practical information as may contribute to the comfort and enjoyment of their sojourn at this beautiful watering-place. Although exhaustive treatises, principally medical, have been written on Carlsbad in other languages, the English contributions to its literature have so far been exceedingly meagre, and have only been obtainable in Carlsbad itself. The present work, therefore, has been undertaken in response to the frequently expressed need of a handbook which intending English and American visitors can consult prior to undertaking the journey, and which it is hoped will prove of practical use during the period of their stay.

We have pleasure in taking this opportunity to tender our grateful acknowledgments to the Burgomeister of Carlsbad, and his courteous secretary, for valuable information received from them during the Author's visit to Carlsbad. We have also to acknowledge our indebtedness to the comprehensive German works on Carlsbad by Dr. Hlawacek, Dr. Rudolf Mannl, Herr Vincenz Prökl, and an excellent *brochure* in French by Dr. W. Pichler, as well as to the admirable articles on Carlsbad, written to the *Times* by its well-known correspondent, Fraser Rae, Esq.

Annexed to the descriptive portion of the work is a medical treatise by Dr. London, resident physician at Carlsbad, which embraces the nature and rules of the treatment, and a synopsis of the various diseases which can be relieved or cured by the use of the Carlsbad waters. Coming from so well-known an authority, this treatise will doubtless be of interest, not only to patients, but also to the medical profession.

CONTENTS.

CARLSBAD AND ITS ENVIRONS.

No.		PAGE
I.	INTRODUCTION	11
	Routes to Carlsbad	19
II.	SITUATION AND CLIMATE	25
III.	HISTORY AND REMINISCENCES OF CARLSBAD	28
IV.	LIFE AT CARLSBAD	48
V.	ARRIVAL, HOTELS, LODGINGS, CAFÉS, AND BEST SHOPS	53
VI.	CONCERTS, THEATRES, AND AMUSEMENTS	59
VII.	TOWN REGULATIONS	62
	Cure and Music Tax	62
	Regulations Respecting Lodgings	64
	Bath Regulations	68
	Public Carriages	72
	Donkeys and Donkey Carriages	76
	Omnibuses	78
	Post and Telegraph Regulations	80
	Dienstmann-Institute	81
VIII.	DESCRIPTION OF THE TOWN AND PRINCIPAL BUILDINGS	83
IX.	THE SPRINGS OF CARLSBAD	93
	Sprudel	97
	Hygiensquelle	99
	Marktbrunn	99
	Kaiser Karlsquelle	100

No.		Page
	Schlossbrunn	100
	Russische Kronequelle	101
	Mühlbrunn	101
	Neubrunn	101
	Bernhardsbrunnen	102
	Elisabethquelle	103
	Felsenquelle	104
	Curhausquelle	105
	Kaiserbrunnen	106
	Eisenquelle	107
	Sauerbrunn	108
X.	WALKS TO THE	
	Alte Wiese, Kiesweg, Posthof, and Kaiser Park	109
	Ecce Homo Kapelle, Franz Josef's Höhe, and Findlater's Temple	114
	Findlater's Pyramid and Freundschafts-Höhe	115
	Hirschensprung	116
	Belvidere and Aberg	118
	Weisses Kreuz and Shützen Park	120
	Panorama, Waldschloss, and Drei Kreuzberg	121
	Wiener Sitz, Sauerbrunn, and Schweizerhof	122
	Schönbrunn	123
	Veitsberg	123
	Rothe-Sauerling	124
	Dallwitz	125
XI.	DRIVES ROUND CARLSBAD—	
	Hammer, Aich, and Hans Heiling-Fels	126
	Engelhaus	130
	Elbogen	137
	Giesshübl-Puchstein	140
	Petschau	144
	Schlaggenwald	145
	Schlackenwerth and Hauenstein	145
	Falkenau	148
	Joachimsthal and the Sonnenwirbel	148

No.		PAGE
	Kupferberg	150
	Fischern, Altrohlau, and Neudeck	151
XII. Longer Excursions—		
	Eger and Marienbad	152
	Frauzensbad	157
	Teplitz	159
XIII. Shooting and Fishing		163
XIV. The Exportation and Products of the Carlsbad Waters		165

MEDICAL TREATISE.

		PAGE
I. Action of the Carlsbad Waters		173
II. Use of the Waters		177
III. External Use of the Waters		179
IV. Dietetics during the Use of the Waters		182
V. General Indications for the Use of the Waters		187
	1. Dyspepsia	188
	2. Gastralgia	189
	3. Dilatation of the Stomach	189
	4. Chronic Catarrh of the Bowels, Chronic Diarrhœa, Chronic Constipation	190
	5. Colic	190
	6. Diseases of the Liver and Biliary Ducts	190
	7. Gallstones and Hepatic Colics	191
	8. Gravel and Small Calculi of the Kidneys and Bladder	192
	9. Gout and Chronic Rheumatism	193
	10. Bright's Disease	194
	11. Diabetes	195
	12. Hæmorrhöids	196
	13. Obesity	196
	14. Prosopalgia and Migraine	196
	15. Diseases of the Sexual System	196
VI. Period at which the Effect of the Waters manifests itself		198

ILLUSTRATIONS.

		PAGE
VIEW OF CARLSBAD	*Facing title*	
STADTPARK		49
GARTENZEILE		83
PARKSTRASSE		85
CURHAUS		89
NEUBAD		93
SPRUDEL COLONNADE		97
MARKTBRUNN		99
MÜHLBRUNN COLONNADE		103
HANS HEILING-FELS		127
ENGELHAUS		131
ELBOGEN		137
GIESSHÜBL-PUCHSTEIN		141
CASTLE OF HAUENSTEIN		145
PLAN OF CARLSBAD AND ENVIRONS	*in packet at end of volume.*	

Part I.

CARLSBAD AND ITS ENVIRONS.

I.

INTRODUCTION.

THE Carlsbad *season* is from the 1st of May to the 1st of September, the most crowded time being from the middle of June till the end of July. The spring at Carlsbad is generally early, and by May the foliage is well advanced, but the weather is apt to be somewhat changeable. Nevertheless the bright sunshine and soft invigorating breezes, so welcome to the invalid after the winter is past; the wild-flowers which grow in the woods and on the hillsides around Carlsbad in such endless variety; the cheerful notes of the feathered songsters as they herald the approaching summer, when their voices will be hushed in the drowsy noon-tide heat; and the first fresh green and the blossoms of the orchards, amply compensate for the few wet days and cloudy skies.

The summers at Carlsbad are generally very warm, but as the life is entirely out of doors, and the walks and resting-places delightfully shaded, the discomforts of the heat are reduced to a minimum, while, to those who are unable to take active exercise, the warm summer days, in which they can remain in the open air without risk of being chilled, are very welcome. But perhaps the pleasantest time of the year at Carlsbad is September and October, when there is little rain, and the air is clear, dry, and bracing, and the tints of the foliage almost rival the brilliant autumn colouring of American woods. The disadvantage, however, of remaining after the 15th September is that the open-air concerts are over and most of the cafés close, although a still considerable number of visitors remain till November. In spite of what several works on Carlsbad, written by Carlsbad physicians and others, say about its advantages as a winter residence, it has no attractions whatever at this season for visitors either sick or well; the hotels are almost all closed; the sole distraction is an occasional concert at the Curhaus; and the ground being generally covered with snow for several months, sometimes to a considerable depth, walking is difficult and unpleasant.

Americans who intend visiting Carlsbad should try and arrange their journey so as to sail from the United States in April, which will secure them time to travel in Europe, after the course of the cure, at the most agreeable season. With the large, fast, and magnificently appointed steamers now crossing the Atlantic, the voyage is no longer to be dreaded, and indeed is exceedingly beneficial to many patients, especially to those suffering from disorders of the liver and stomach, or from lung complaints. The enforced relaxation from

I.

INTRODUCTION.

THE Carlsbad *season* is from the 1st of May to the 1st of September, the most crowded time being from the middle of June till the end of July. The spring at Carlsbad is generally early, and by May the foliage is well advanced, but the weather is apt to be somewhat changeable. Nevertheless the bright sunshine and soft invigorating breezes, so welcome to the invalid after the winter is past; the wildflowers which grow in the woods and on the hillsides around Carlsbad in such endless variety; the cheerful notes of the feathered songsters as they herald the approaching summer, when their voices will be hushed in the drowsy noon-tide heat; and the first fresh green and the blossoms of the orchards, amply compensate for the few wet days and cloudy skies.

The summers at Carlsbad are generally very warm, but as the life is entirely out of doors, and the walks and resting-places delightfully shaded, the discomforts of the heat are reduced to a minimum, while, to those who are unable to take active exercise, the warm summer days, in which they can remain in the open air without risk of being chilled, are very welcome. But perhaps the pleasantest time of the year at Carlsbad is September and October, when there is little rain, and the air is clear, dry, and bracing, and the tints of the foliage almost rival the brilliant autumn colouring of American woods. The disadvantage, however, of remaining after the 15th September is that the open-air concerts are over and most of the cafés close, although a still considerable number of visitors remain till November. In spite of what several works on Carlsbad, written by Carlsbad physicians and others, say about its advantages as a winter residence, it has no attractions whatever at this season for visitors either sick or well; the hotels are almost all closed; the sole distraction is an occasional concert at the Curhaus; and the ground being generally covered with snow for several months, sometimes to a considerable depth, walking is difficult and unpleasant.

Americans who intend visiting Carlsbad should try and arrange their journey so as to sail from the United States in April, which will secure them time to travel in Europe, after the course of the cure, at the most agreeable season. With the large, fast, and magnificently appointed steamers now crossing the Atlantic, the voyage is no longer to be dreaded, and indeed is exceedingly beneficial to many patients, especially to those suffering from disorders of the liver and stomach, or from lung complaints. The enforced relaxation from daily business anxieties during the voyage is also of great value to business men, in affording them an opportunity of banishing from their minds the cares they have left behind them.

The present travel across the Atlantic has reached such large proportions that, in spite of the number of steamers sailing weekly, the best state-rooms are generally engaged months ahead; American travellers are therefore strongly advised not to leave engaging their rooms till near the time of sailing. The seasons the steamers are most crowded are, from America, during the spring and early summer months, and from England, during the late summer and autumn months. If the intending traveller be not a good sailor, he should secure a berth as nearly amidships as possible, preferring the bow to the stern. This is a matter of the utmost importance, as the most trying hour on board ship is when dressing in the morning, and it will often depend on the situation of the state-room whether the passenger comes through it safely or not. In rough weather the difference between the motion at the bow or stern, and amidships is very marked indeed. As so much of the comfort at sea, therefore, depends upon having a well-situated state-room, it is advisable, if possible, to go over the ship and see the position of the state-room before engaging it. Nervous invalids should not take their state-rooms near the pantry, as the clatter of the dishes is very disturbing; they should also, if possible, avoid the proximity of the cinder-shoot from the engine-room. Invalids should also choose the sunny side of the ship.

Useful Hints for the Passage.—Travellers are recommended to get a steamer trunk or bag that will fit under the berth, to contain the articles required on the passage; the space between the floor and bottom of lower berth is generally about 15 inches. We also strongly recommend getting a "steamer chair," which will be found most useful on the voyage, especially if the weather be at all fine; a good supply of rugs and shawls should also be taken. All the steamers have bath-rooms, and those who desire their morning "tub" should, as soon as coming on board, register their name and the time at which they would like to take their bath with the barber or bath-room steward (whoever has charge of the baths), as the demand for the baths generally exceeds the supply. Travellers making the passage across the Atlantic who are liable to sea-sickness will do well not to put their trust in any of the so-called remedies for sea-sickness. Some of these may alleviate the trouble on a short passage, but no remedy, except that of becoming accustomed to the motion of the vessel, will cure sea-sickness on an Atlantic voyage, and the best thing the unfortunate sufferer can do is to brace up as well as he can, be as much as possible on deck, and live plainly; and, from long experience, we can assure timid travellers that it is very rarely *mal-de-mer* lasts more than the first day or two. The purser allots the places at table. The usual fees on board the

Atlantic steamers are 10s. each to the table and bed-room stewards, and 2s. 6d. to the "boots;" or in the case of ladies, 10s. to the stewardess who attends to the ladies' state-rooms. A collection is also made among the frequenters of the smoking-room for the smoking-room steward.

The meals on board are usually:—Breakfast between 8.30 and 10 A.M.; lunch, 1 P.M.; dinner, 6 P.M.

Invalids going to Carlsbad can save the fatiguing part of the journey from Liverpool to Germany, and the discomforts of crossing the Channel, by taking one of the fine new steamers "Elbe," "Werra," "Fulda," "Ems," or "Eider," of the North German Lloyd, to Bremen. The appointments of these steamers are fully equal to any of the Liverpool lines, while the *cuisine* is superior.

General Hints.—We cannot do better than preface these remarks with the excellent advice of Dr. E. Gutmann, the well-known authority on European spas, "that patients in the last stage of consumption or Bright's disease, or other chronic affections, should not be allowed to undergo the hardships and the excitement of a trip to a watering-place, thereby sacrificing the little amount of strength they still possess for the imaginary hope of an impossible cure. It is the sacred duty of the physician to dissuade them from the journey, though very often the contrary takes place. Every bath physician during the bath season has the opportunity of examining quite a number of incurable invalids, who have been sent to the spa by unscrupulous medical advisers, never again to return to their homes. Far away from their families, surrounded by strangers, more helpless and suffering than ever before, they vainly long for the tender care of their relatives during the last days of their earthly pilgrimage."

It should not be forgotten that the waters of Carlsbad are powerful remedies, and no invalid should go there without having first consulted his own physician and obtained from him a certificate stating the history and nature of his disease, which he should hand to the physician at Carlsbad under whose care he intends placing himself. This will save the bath physician much time and trouble, and enable him to prescribe the treatment at Carlsbad with greater certainty. The *usual* stay is four weeks; but it is quite impossible even for an experienced physician to accurately determine beforehand how long it will be necessary for a patient to take the waters, and indeed it is often the case that a patient must return for two or three consecutive years before a radical cure can be effected.

Having chosen his route, the invalid should proceed by short and easy stages, and should by all means avoid travelling at night, which on the Continent, with the exception of the few lines which run *wagons-lits*, is most uncomfortable. For the convenience of travellers we append to the routes to Carlsbad a list of the most interesting places on the way, with the principal sights and best hotel at each.

On all Continental lines the amount of the fare is stamped on the tickets. The fare should be tendered in the coin of the country, and not in English bank notes or gold, as the rate of exchange at the railway stations will sometimes be found anything but satisfactory. The change should always be counted.

The second class carriages in Germany and Austria are comfortable, and are used by a most respectable class of travellers, and, except for invalids who may wish to have as few fellow-travellers as possible, the small extra comfort of the first class is hardly worth the additional cost. In France, however, the second class carriages generally speaking are uncomfortable, and certainly quite unsuited for ladies or invalids. In travelling from Paris, or any other place in France, to any place in Germany and Austria by the express trains, the traveller can purchase a *mixed ticket* entitling him to travel first class to the frontier, and thence to his destination in the second class.

As the trains in the Continent seldom wait long enough at the stations to give time for a meal, a luncheon basket should always be taken.

When circular or through tickets are taken the ticket must be stamped at the ticket office, both on arrival and departure, when the journey is broken at any intermediate station.

Travellers should always be careful to see that the

B

conductor when collecting the ticket tears out the proper coupon.

In Germany and Austria smoking is permitted in all carriages except those marked 'Nicht Raucher,' and in compartments reserved for ladies. In France compartments are set apart for travellers who wish to smoke (marked 'Fumeurs'); and no smoking is allowed in any other except with the consent of the occupants. The guard will always interfere to prevent smoking in the non-smoking compartments if he is requested to do so. Lavatories and other conveniences, 'cabinets ambulants,' are attached to most of the express trains.

With regard to luggage, on the ocean steamers no limit is made, and whatever may be the printed rules of the steamship companies on the subject, practically, the traveller is permitted to carry all the personal luggage he may desire. In France and Belgium 56 lbs. of luggage per passenger is carried free, but on the Rhine railways, and on most of the German lines, a charge is made for all luggage except such as is taken in the carriage. The charge for extra luggage on the Continent is very high, and if the visitor to Carlsbad intends taking a quantity of luggage with him, considerable expense may be saved by sending it on by goods trains through some express company. Baggage forwarded in this way, however, should be sent on at least a week in advance.

English bank notes and gold can be exchanged everywhere on the Continent. The rate of exchange is generally 25 francs, 20 marks, or 12 Austrian florins to the pound, but a little more than this can be obtained at respectable banks or exchange offices. English silver is of no use except at a very low exchange.

As the weather of Carlsbad is liable to sudden changes, visitors should be provided with both warm and light clothing. It is not necessary for invalids to encumber their luggage with a number of "invalid comforts," such as English tea, biscuits, &c., as they can be obtained at Carlsbad. Smokers, however, who are particular, should take their cigars, cigarettes, and tobacco, although they will find when they have paid the duty they will have become somewhat expensive.

Routes to Carlsbad.

The two main routes from London to Carlsbad are—

(1.) *Via* Brussels, Cologne, Mayence, Aschaffenburg, and Eger. Between Aschaffenburg and Eger some of the trains run *via* Nuremberg, and others *via* Bamberg and Oberkotzau. Travellers intending to go through without stopping will find this the quickest and most direct route.

(2.) *Via* Paris, Strassburg, Carlsruhe, Stuttgart, Nuremberg, and Eger.

The length of the journey, of course, depends upon the length of the stoppages made by the way, but the time consumed in actual travelling is about one and a half days *via* Calais or Ostend.

The best train from London *via* Calais and Ostend is the 8 P.M., as it gives an opportunity of travelling up the Rhine by daylight.

If the journey to Brussels is taken by the London, Chatham, and Dover service, *via* Queenborough and Flushing, or by the Great Eastern service, *via* Harwich and Rotterdam or Antwerp, the time is about four to six hours longer. The steamers on both these services are large, swift, and exceedingly comfortable, and the fares about twenty shillings cheaper.

The night express trains from Calais, Ostend, Flushing, Rotterdam, and Antwerp to Cologne have sleeping carriages. Travellers from Paris can take the *Orient Express*, leaving in the evening, as far as Stuttgart, where it arrives about nine o'clock the next morning. This train, which is exceedingly comfortable, is composed entirely of sleeping, dining, and drawing-room carriages. The fares are about 25 per cent. more than by the ordinary expresses, but to those who can afford it, the additional comfort is well worth the extra charge.

Carlsbad can also be reached from Paris by Strassburg, Appenweier, Heidelberg, and Aschaffenburg (see above). Also by Pagny-sur-Moselle, Forbach, Bingerbruck, Mayence, and Aschaffenburg (see above). These routes take from four to six hours longer than the route *via* Stuttgart.

(3.) An exceedingly pleasant and interesting route to Carlsbad, though somewhat longer and more expensive than the above routes, is from Paris to Bâle, thence to Zurich and Rorschach, across the Lake of Constance by steamer to Lindau, thence to Munich, Pilsen, and Carlsbad.

Note.—Through tickets are only issued from London by Route I.

Routes from London.	Fares.			
	Single Tickets.		Return Tickets, available for 30 days.	
	1st Cl.	2nd Cl.	1st Cl.	2nd Cl.
	£ s. d.	£ s. d.	£ s. d.	£ s. d.
Harwich, Rotterdam, Cologne, Mayence, Wurzburg, Nuremburg, Eger	5 16 3	4 3 7	10 14 9	7 14 8
Queenboro', Flushing, Cologne, Mayence, &c., as above	6 2 7	4 9 0	10 18 0	7 18 6
Harwich, Antwerp, Brussels, Cologne, Mayence, &c., as above . . .	5 17 0	4 3 0	10 10 6	7 10 0
Dover, Calais (or Ostend), Brussels, &c., as above .	6 17 0	5 0 0	11 17 6	8 15 3

The fares *via* Paris are about £7, 10s. first class, and £5, 5s. second class.

PRINCIPAL PLACES OF INTEREST ON THE ABOVE ROUTES.

ROUTE I.

Brussels.—Hôtel Mengelle. Sights: Cathedral of St. Guduld, Hôtel de Ville, King's Palace, Museums, Zoological Gardens, Wiertz Museum, Gallery of the Duke of Arenberg, the New Palais de Justice, and the Bois de Cambre.

Aix-la-Chapelle.—Hôtel Grand Monarque. Sights: Cathedral, Rathaus, Elisenbrunnen, Kurhaus, Suermondt Museum, and Lousberg.

Cologne.—Hôtel du Nord. Sights: Cathedral, Wallraf-Richartz Museum, Episcopal Museum, Rathaus, Gürzenich, Churches of St. Gereon, St. Maria-im-Capitol, and St. Ursula, Monument of Frederick William III., Flora and Zoological Gardens.

Coblenz.—Hôtel du Géant. Sights: Fortress of Ehrenbreitstein, Rhine Promenade, Church of St. Castor, The Castor Brunnen, The Burg, Kaufhaus, Moselle Bridge, Imperial Palace, The Petersberg.

Mayence.—Hôtel de Hollande. Sights: Cathedral, Gutenberg Monument, The Citadel and Eigelstein, Museum in the Palace, New Promenade on the Rhine.

Frankfort.—Hôtel Schwan. Sights: The Kaisersaal in the Römer, Cathedral, Ariadneum, Picture Galleries of the Städel Institute, Kunst Verein, and Kunstgewerbe-Verein, Historical Museum, Jenkenberg Natural History Museum, New Opera, Zoological Garden, Palm Garden.

Würzberg.—Hôtel Kronprinz. Sights: Cathedral, Neue Münster, Royal Palace, Marien Kapelle, Citadel.

Nuremberg.—Hôtel de Bavière. Sights: Church of St. Lawrence, Frauen Kirche, Rathaus, Church of St. Sebaldus, Schöne Brunnen, Germanic Museum, The Burg.

Route II.

Strasburg.—Hôtel de la Ville de Paris. Sights: Cathedral, Church of St. Thomas, Statue of Gutenberg, The Broglie.

Stuttgart.—Hôtel Marquardt. Sights: Königs Bau, New Palace, Old Palace, Stifts Kirche, Natural History Museum, Museum of Art, Stadt Garten, and Anlagen.

Route III.

Bâle.—Hôtel Trois Rois. Sights: Cathedral, Cathedral Museum, Rathaus, Town Museum, Zoological Garden.

Zurich.—Hôtel Bauer au Lac. Sights: Stadt Garten, Stadthaus, Grossmunster, St. Peter's Church, Wasser Kirche, The Tonhalle, Höhe Promenade, Town Museum, Kunster Gütli Museum, The Arsenal, Botanic Garden, Excursion to the Uetliberg.

Munich.—Hotel Four Seasons. Sights: Royal Palace, Alte Pinakothek, Glyptothek, Neue Pinakothek, National Museum, The Basilica, Count Schäck's Picture Gallery, The Propylæa, Monument of Maximilian II., Mariahilf Kirche, Royal Library, Hof Garten, Aquarium, Hall of Fame and Statue of Bavaria, English Garden.

TABLE OF MONEY, WEIGHTS, AND MEASURES.

American.		English.			French, Swiss, or Italian.		German.		Austrian.		
Dols.	*cents.*	*£*	*s.*	*d.*	*Frs.*	*centms.*	*Marks.*	*Pf.*	*Florins.*	*Kr.*	
0	1	0	0	0½	0	5	0	4	0	2½	approximate
0	5	0	0	2½	0	25	0	20	0	10	
0	10	0	0	5	0	50	0	40	0	25¾	
0	20	0	0	9¾	1	0	0	80	0	51	
0	25	0	1	0	1	25	1	0	0	60	
0	50	0	2	0	2	50	2	0	1	20	
1	0	0	4	0	5	0	4	0	2	40	
4	86	1	0	0	25	20	20	30	12	55	actual

(The Austrian gulden or florin equals 1*s.* 8*d.* English money.)

Weights (Approximate).

1 Gramme = 1/28 oz.
1 Hectogramme = 3½ oz.
1 Kilogramme = 2⅕ lbs.
51 Kilogrammes = 1 cwt.
1015 Kilogrammes = 1 ton.

Linear Measures.

1 Centimètre = ⅖ inch.
1 Mètre = 3 ft. 3¼ inches.
1 Kilomètre = ⅝ mile.
8 Kilomètres = 5 miles.

Land Measures.

1 Centiare = 1⅕ sq. yd.
1 Are = ¼ acre.
1 Hectare = 2½ acres.

Fluid Measures.

1 Litre = 1¾ pints.
4½ Litres = 1 gallon.
1 Hectolitre = 22 gallons.

THERMOMETER.

Far.	Cent.	Réaumur.	Far.	Cent.	Réaumur.	Far.	Cent.	Réaumur.	Far.	Cent.	Réaumur.
104°	40°	32°	77°	25°	24°	55°	13°	10°	37°	3°	2°
98	37	29	76	24	19	50	10	8	35	1·25	1
95	35	28	68	20	16	41	5	4	33	1	0·8
86	30	24	59	15	12	39	4	3	32	0	0·0

II.

SITUATION AND CLIMATE.

CARLSBAD, one of the most attractive and beautiful of European watering-places, is situated in the north-west of Bohemia, in lat. 50° and long. 13°. The town lies in the narrow and winding valley of the Tepel, near its junction with the Eger, 1124 feet above the level of the sea. On either side of the valley rise picturesque and rugged hills of volcanic formation, the highest of which, called the Ewige Leben, or 'Eternal Life,' is 2003 feet above the sea-level, or 879 feet above the town. These hills are covered with woods of pine, spruce, beech, elm, birch, and oak; spruce and pine predominating. Numberless paths intersect the woods in all directions, affording shady and picturesque walks, and on the level portion of the valley, and over some of the gentler slopes, are well-kept carriage roads. The composition of these hills is of three varieties of granite: gneiss, quartz, and argillaceous schist, the rocks being intersected with the usual fissures accompanying this formation. On some of the hills are strata and out-croppings of basalt, and extensive veins of hornstone.

A humorist has said that Carlsbad "is built on the lid of a boiling kettle," which is almost literally true, as it stands on a crust of comparative thinness, through which rise no less than nineteen springs of various temperatures. Borings which have been made in the crust have reached a vast and seething subterranean cauldron below, of immeasurable depth. This crust, on which the Marktplatz, the Kreuzgasse, and the Mühlbrunn Colonnade are built, is mostly composed of Sprudelstein, or Sprudelschelle (Sprudel-stone or Sprudel-shell), a hard stone, capable of taking a fine polish. The Sprudelstein is supposed to have been formed by the mineral constituents of the springs being gradually deposited as they came into contact with the open air (see page 95).

THE CLIMATE of Carlsbad, like that of all mountainous districts, is rather changeable, but the air is remarkably pure and invigorating, the town never having been visited by any contagious diseases or epidemics. It entirely escaped the Pest of the Middle Ages, and during the Austro-German war, when cholera, brought by the sick and wounded soldiers, was raging in the surrounding districts, not a single case occurred at Carlsbad. There is no stagnant water in the neighbourhood, and consequently malaria is unknown. In summer, even when the days are very warm, the nights and early mornings are generally cool and invigorating. Owing to the character of its soil, which permits of moisture being rapidly absorbed, the roads and paths around Carlsbad become perfectly dry, and are fit for walking in a few hours, after even heavy rain. The mean temperature of the year is $43\frac{1}{2}°$ Fahr.; in summer, $66\frac{1}{2}°$ Fahr.; in spring and autumn, $47°$ Fahr.; and in winter $27\frac{7}{10}°$ Fahr. The prevailing winds are from the west and north, the latter of which, having free access to the town, is generally cool and bracing.

III.

HISTORY AND REMINISCENCES OF CARLSBAD.

CARLSBAD is one of the very few important European watering-places which does not appear to have been known to the Romans. The town was originally incorporated by King John of Luxemburg, who, by an ancient charter dated 1325, conferred on it certain rights and privileges, though there is no doubt from the name, *Wary*, or 'Warm,' that the hot springs were known long before this period.

The discovery of the springs is traditionally attributed to the Emperor Charles IV., son of King John, who in the year 1358 was hunting in the neighbourhood while on a visit to the castle of Elbogen (see page 137). One of his dogs while following a wounded deer fell over a cliff, since called the 'Hirschensprung,' or Deer's Leap (see page 116), into one of the hot springs below. Attracted by its cries, the hunters came to the rescue of the animal, and on taking it out, found it severely wounded by its fall. Its subsequent recovery was so rapid, that the Emperor's physician attributed it to the healing power of the water, and he induced his royal master, who was suffering from an old wound in his leg, received at the battle of Crecy, to test its efficacy. The Emperor's wound also rapidly healed, and in gratitude he founded a town at the springs and named it Carlsbad.

As, however, the existence of the springs was known long before this time, the legend, as far as their first discovery is concerned, is purely mythical, though the incident itself may actually have occurred. But if the Emperor did not first discover Carlsbad, he gave it its present name, extended the charter granted by King John, and built a royal residence in the town.

Of the early history of Carlsbad we have no certain data, as the archives of the town were almost entirely destroyed by fire in 1604. In the middle of the sixth century the Eger district was settled by a horde of Slavs, who came from the plains of Russia and Lithuania, and from whom the present Bohemian people are descended. These Slavs were pagans, and it was not until after Bohemia was united to the German Empire by Charlemagne in A.D. 800, that Christianity began to spread among them; indeed, paganism did not finally disappear till the tenth century. In the ninth century the district of Eger came into possession of the powerful Margrave Vohburg, who built the castle of Elbogen in 870, and it seems impossible that the remarkable phenomena of the hot springs should have been unknown to those who lived so near them. A chronicle written about this time mentions the rivers Tepel and Eger, which in the original Slav language meant 'tepid' and 're-warmed.' Another curious fact is that the walls of the castle of Neudeck, built at the commencement of the thirteenth century, and distant about nine miles from Carlsbad, are partly constructed of Sprudelstone.

In 1149 the whole of the Eger district, together with the towns of Falkenau, Elbogen, and Warmbad (or *Wary*), became the personal property of the German Emperor, Frederick Barbarossa, who received it as a dowry on his marriage with Adelheid, daughter of the Margrave Diebold von Vohburg.

The nomenclature of the towns and villages which were founded before the commencement of the twelfth century is almost entirely Slavonic; the settlements founded after the district came into possession of the Emperor Frederick Barbarossa in 1149 having been generally given German names. We may, therefore, assume that the towns, and villages, and castles with Bohemian names were founded before, and those with German, founded after this date.

In 1306 John of Luxemburg, the blind King who was killed at the battle of Crecy in 1349, was elected King of Bohemia, and in 1317 he visited the castle of Elbogen (see page 137) with his consort and his infant son. In 1325, by a charter which still exists, he enfiefed the town and granted it certain privileges, which he increased by a second charter dated 1337. In 1358 the Emperor Charles IV., son of King John, built a royal castle at Carlsbad, at which time the town consisted of only forty houses, and in 1370 granted a new charter, conferring on the citizens rights of self-government and the free choice of magistrates. A transcript of this charter, in which *Wary* is first called *Carlsbad*, still exists. Charles died in 1378, and his son, Wencelaus I., confirmed all these privileges. At the end of the fourteenth or beginning of the fifteenth centuries the estate of Elbogen, with Carlsbad, was separated from the district of Eger, and came into possession of the Bohemian royal family; how, is not exactly known, but the first step which led to this was doubtless the foreclosing of a mortgage of 7000 marks silver, which Wencelaus I. claimed had been lent by his father, Charles IV., to the heirs of Frederick Barbarossa.

An eventful period in the history of Carlsbad commences with the mortgaging in 1434 of the Burgravate of Elbogen by the crown to the Chancellor Caspar Schlick for 11,900 florins. Schlick had constant feuds with a neighbouring magnate, Count Von Eulenburg, who, in the prosecution of certain personal claims he had against the Chancellor, made frequent raids on Carlsbad and the Elbogen district, burning the houses and plundering the inhabitants. These outrages were returned in kind by Schlick and his followers, till they reached such a height that the German Parliament in 1444 passed a special Act for their suppression. In 1455 Heronimus Schlick, the nephew of Caspar, mortgaged the castle of Carlsbad to Count Polaczky von Polaky for 500 florins, reserving to himself the protectorate of the town. A feud soon broke out between these nobles; the citizens of Elbogen siding with Schlick, and those of Carlsbad taking the part of Polaky. In one of their numerous fights Polaky took 200 of the Elbogeners prisoners and brought them to the castle at Carlsbad, which was, however, shortly afterwards besieged and taken by Schlick, and the prisoners set at liberty. This feud was finally settled by arbitration, and three umpires were appointed by King Wladislaw, the decision being that Schlick had to pay to Polaky 600 florins to redeem his debt, and receive back his castle at Carlsbad.

In 1462 civil war broke out in Bohemia owing to the issue of a Papal bull by Pope Pius forbidding the taking of the wine at the sacrament by laymen. King George of Bohemia, on his refusal to allow his subjects to obey the bull, was deposed by the Pope, who offered the crown to King Matthias Corvinus of Hungary. The greater part of Bohemia rebelled and went over to King Matthias, but a still influential number of his subjects, among whom were the Burgrave Schlick and his vassals of Elbogen and Carlsbad, remained faithful for a time. Owing, however, to the rapidly increasing power of King Matthias and the persuasions of Papal emissaries, together with threats of excommunication from Rome, they finally deserted their sovereign, and sent him a letter renouncing their allegiance. After the restoration of peace on the death of George, the Burgrave Matthias Schlick commenced to plunder and oppress the citizens of Elbogen and Carlsbad, and succeeded in making himself so unpopular that he lost all control over his followers. Schlick vainly appealed to King Matthias for assistance to quell the insurrection, and finding himself unable to cope with his rebellious vassals, he made over the Burgravate of Elbogen and Carlsbad in 1470 to the brothers, Elector Ernst and Duke Albrecht of Saxony, for the sum of 23,000 florins. The Elbogeners, however, relished as little the rule of their new masters as of their former ruler, and declined to take the oath of allegiance. The brothers took up arms in 1471, and laid siege to the castle of Elbogen, which was surrendered by treachery, and numbers of its defenders were hung over the castle walls. After the subjugation of the Elbogeners peace was concluded, Schlick being permitted to remain actual lord in fief, while Duke Albrecht became lord protector. No sooner, however, was Schlick reinstated than he began a second time to harass and oppress the citizens of Elbogen and Carlsbad, and on their again showing signs of rebellion he arranged with Duke Albrecht to make another raid on Elbogen. This plan was executed on the night of the 1st October 1476; the town was taken and plundered, and frightful atrocities were committed by Schlick and his followers, in consequence of which many of the citizens emigrated.

For the next fifty years the history of the town is simply one of petty feuds and personal quarrels.

In 1480 we have the first mention of a 'Cur-guest,' Fräulein Barbara Schenk von Frautenburg, who came for the cure accompanied by her mother.

In 1531 Albert Schlick, grandson of Matthias, founded in Carlsbad a hospital for indigent patients, which he dedicated to the Holy Spirit. He also obtained a charter from King Wladislaw giving him the right to exact from all visitors to Carlsbad, rich or poor, a donation for the hospital; the amount being left to the guests themselves. This was the first 'Cur-tax' imposed at Carlsbad.

In 1533 Albert Schlick exchanged with his cousin, Hermonius, the Burgravate of Elbogen and Carlsbad for that of Winteritz. On the outbreak of the war between Bohemia and Saxony, Hermonius Schlick renounced his allegiance to his sovereign and joined the Saxon army. After the disastrous defeat of the Saxons at the battle of Muhlberg, 24th April 1547, Hermonius was outlawed, but on the conclusion of peace he managed to obtain a pardon from the Emperor Ferdinand I., his estates of Elbogen and Carlsbad, however, being confiscated to the crown. The town of Carslbad was then incorporated and made a royal borough, and the citizens took the oath of allegiance to Ferdinand.

There being now no resident Burgrave, the castle of Carlsbad for a long time remained unoccupied, and the citizens not wishing to see this historic building fall into decay, petitioned the Emperor

Maximilian to make it over to the town for the use of the fire-brigade. This request was granted by a deed dated 1567.

The crown still retained possession of all the land and other property attached to the Burgravate of Carlsbad, and the citizens for many years tried in vain to acquire them. They, however, succeeded at last in purchasing them from the needy Emperor Rudolph in 1598 for the sum of 52,800 marks. By this purchase the town gained considerably, and also greatly extended its influence and status.

When the Reformation began to spread in Bohemia at the commencement of the sixteenth century, the then reigning Burgrave, Sebastian Schlick, who was a friend of Luther, energetically devoted himself to furthering the cause of the new faith, and succeeded in establishing the Protestant religion throughout the whole Eger district. The first Reformed preacher, Wolfgang Rappold, was appointed in Elbogen in 1523. A Lutheran pastor was doubtless appointed about the same time to Carlsbad, though the first reference made in existing records is to the preaching of Andreas Hampisch in the Andreas Church in 1554. After the death of the Emperor Rudolph in 1612, his successor, Ferdinand II., who was bitterly opposed to the Reformed faith, re-established the Catholic religion throughout Bohemia, and in 1624 the parish church of Carlsbad was again made over to the Romanists, in consequence of which the last Lutheran pastor, Johann Georg Kreizel, together with a large number of the citizens, emigrated to Saxony and founded the town of Johanngeorgenstadt. On the Galgenburg, above the Chapel of St. Mary, is a large stone which commemorates this exodus.

During the Thirty Years' War Carlsbad suffered severely, the town being repeatedly sacked, and many of the citizens killed.

The fame of Carlsbad as a resort for crowned heads and personages of the highest rank dates from the visit of the Archduke Ferdinand in 1571, who was accompanied by his consort, Philippina Welser, the daughter of an Augsburg merchant, who won all hearts, even of the Archduke's royal relations, by her beauty and accomplishments.

In 1630 Carlsbad was visited by Wallenstein, Duke of Friedland, who was afterwards barbarously murdered in the Castle of Eger (see page 153).

In 1683 the Crown Prince of Saxony, afterwards George III., with the Duke of Lauenburg, came to Carlsbad for the cure, accompanied with a large retinue, and stayed six weeks. During their visit they gave great entertainments, at one of which, we are told, an ox stuffed with capons was roasted whole and served in the Fest Platz, now occupied by the garden of the Hotel Goldener Schild. All the inhabitants of the town were summoned to the banquet by a fanfare of trumpets and kettledrums stationed on the Hirschensprung. The Prince, dressed in a servant's livery of red and green, waited on the guests himself. The festivities wound up with a ball, the music being supplied by an orchestra of fiddles, pipes, and steinbok horns!

In 1691 Augustus I., King of Poland, accompanied by the famous beauty, Aurora, Countess von Königstein, took the cure at Carlsbad. He was accompanied by so many soldiers that temporary barracks had to be erected for their accommodation in the fields. He entertained the visitors and townspeople with tournaments on the Alte Wiese, and on the Allée Platz he gave a grand entertainment in a ballroom he had erected, and decorated with Bohemian lustres and mirrors. We are told he provided a surprise for his guests by having the water from the Sprudel conducted in pipes to the ballroom, and while the ball was at its height he had the water turned on and gave the dancers a thorough drenching.

At this time the Cur-guests at Carlsbad were such insatiate pleasure-seekers that, in addition to the almost nightly *fêtes*, they had *matinées dansantes* every day from 11 A.M. to 1 P.M.

The years 1711 and 1712 were memorable from the visits of Peter the Great, who came to be cured of rheumatism.

We are told that the Czar on his arrival was ordered by his physician to take three glasses of the waters before breakfast, but by some misunderstanding he thought three large pitchers were meant. He managed to get down one, and was almost choking over the second, when the doctor, fortunately appearing, informed him of his mistake. He must, besides this, have swallowed a considerable quantity of the waters during his stay, as he was in the habit of taking twenty-three glasses at a time.

In a letter dated 19th September, written to the Empress Catherine, he says: "We, thank God, are well, only our bellies are swelled up with water, because we drink like horses, and have nothing else to do." In the following year he writes again to his wife: "We began to drink the waters at this hole yesterday. How it works I will write, but don't look for any other news from this wilderness." The treatment may have benefited him in a bodily sense, but it certainly did not improve his violent temper. We are told that he took part in the annual shooting match at Carlsbad, and carried off the prize. One of the spectators, whose admiration had been excited by his fine shooting, began to vigorously applaud, when the Czar, thinking he was trying to distract his aim, fired at him, but fortunately missed him. On another occasion he assisted at the building of a house, laying the stones with his own hands. One of the masons, who was gazing at him in astonishment, was the victim of a similar outbreak of temper. One of the peculiarities of the Czar was an intense dislike of being watched while he was at work, and on seeing the mason looking at him he became so enraged that he threw a trowelful of mortar in his face. On finding his mistake, however, he made ample amends in both cases by apologising and presenting the men with handsome sums of money. There being no

Russian church at Carlsbad, the Czar went daily to offer up his prayers before the cross on the Hirschensprung, on the spot since named the Petershöhe (see page 117).

At the shooting match referred to, the Czar had given as the prize, a cask of wine, which had been sent him by the Emperor Charles VI., and on winning it himself he refused to take it back. Another contest was therefore held, in which the Czar did not compete. The winner of the cask at the second contest had it bottled in small flasks which readily sold at a high price, and invested the proceeds for the benefit of the shooting society, to whom this fund still yields an income of thirty florins a year. The target which the Czar shot at is preserved in the Schiesshaus.

It was at Carlsbad that Peter carried on the negotiations for the marriage of his son Alexis with the Princess Charlotte of Wolfenbüttel, whom the Prince first met at the Castle of Schlackenwerth. It was at first proposed that the marriage should take place secretly at Carlsbad, but it was eventually solemnised at Dresden. The Czar left Carlsbad to attend the marriage, contrary to the advice of his physicians, which led to his experiencing a serious relapse. During his second visit to Carlsbad in 1712 Peter renewed his acquaintance with the celebrated philosopher Leibnitz, whose advice received at that time proved of such assistance to the Czar in introducing reforms into Russia. The Czar lived in the house 'Zum Rothen Herz,' on the Alte Wiese.

In the same year, 1712, the Empress Christina of Austria, with a large retinue, visited Carlsbad, accompanied by her daughter, the Princess Maria Theresa, then four years of age. In honour of her visit the citizens had a beautiful drinking goblet made for her at the famous porcelain manufactory at Meissen. This goblet is now in the museum at Prague.

In 1732 Carlsbad was honoured with a visit from the Emperor Charles II. and his consort, the Empress Christina, who seem to have been accompanied by about half the nobility of Austria. The town records of that time relate that it required 6600 horses to convey their Majesties and their retinue to the place. The Emperor during his stay took a great interest in Carlsbad. He rebuilt the parish church, and gave largely to the charities and for improving the town.

During the war of succession, which broke out after the ascent of Maria Theresa to the throne of Austria in 1740, Carlsbad suffered severely, as well as Eger and Elbogen, these three towns being sacked by the French and the citizens laid under heavy contribution.

In 1762 the first Cur-lists were published. These lists were in writing, the first printed lists not being published till 1794.

In 1766 commenced what may be termed a new era in the history of Carlsbad, as in that year the celebrated physician, Dr. David Becher, made the first scientific analysis of the medical and chemical properties of the waters, and laid down regulations for their use which were practically the same as those in force to-day, and which have proved so beneficial to hundreds of thousands of patients for the last century. From this time the number of visitors has steadily increased;—from 445 in 1785 to 28,600 in 1885. This rapid increase encouraged the municipal authorities to provide better accommodation for visitors, and to take steps for making the town more attractive. Fine chestnut alleys were planted and walks were laid out along the Tepel and through the woods. In 1774 a new drinking and bathing hall was erected in place of the old Sprudel Hall.

One of the most celebrated leaders of Carlsbad society at this period was Count Maurice von Brühl, the intimate friend of Admiral Orloff (see page 114). At one of the great open-air *fêtes* he gave on the Plobensberg fresh flowers were fastened to the trees in the woods, which gave them the appearance of a forest in bloom.

In 1784 the municipality erected the fine stone bridge over the Eger which now leads to the railway station.

In 1794 the "Sprudel Book," in which all visitors entered their voluntary contributions, was abolished, and an act was passed ordering that every nobleman should pay a cur-tax of two florins, and every commoner one florin. In 1800 the walls which confine the course of the Tepel were built, and a row of wooden booths or shops erected along the 'Alte Wiese.' At this time Carlsbad benefited greatly from the visits of Lord Findlater, a Scotch nobleman, who, in gratitude for the great benefit he derived from drinking the waters, gave large sums of money to the local charities and for laying out and beautifying the environs of the town.

In 1785, when thirty-four years of age, Goethe paid his first visit to Carlsbad, where he afterwards spent many of the happiest and most fruitful years of his life. He altogether paid fourteen visits to Carlsbad, and there is little doubt but that the drinking of the waters greatly contributed to prolong his life and added greatly to his vigour of both mind and body. The houses in the Markt Platz in which he lived are marked by marble tablets. Goethe from his youth was afflicted with a painful malady which caused himself and his friends great anxiety. After much suffering he was at last persuaded to try the efficacy of the Carlsbad waters. Shortly after his first arrival in 1785 he wrote that he had already experienced great benefit, and that pleasant intercourse with the visitors had "rubbed off the rust" he had gathered in the retired life he had hitherto been obliged to lead. A touching incident is related of his visit in 1819. "The 28th August being his seventieth birthday, the Grand Duke of Mecklenburg provided a pleasant and most agreeable surprise for him by bringing the old clock which hung up in the house where he first saw the light and spent his youth at Frankfort, and having it hung up in his Carlsbad lodgings. When Goethe awoke early in the morning and heard the clock strike the hour, he called to his servant, saying, 'I hear a clock strike that arouses all the memories of my childhood. Is it a dream or a reality?' Then he got up, and learning the truth, was moved to tears." His last visit was in 1823. He was then seventy-four, but, susceptible as ever, he fell in love with a charming young lady, Fräulein von Levetzov. He proposed marriage, which she declined, although she never married afterwards, and when the bust of the poet was unveiled in 1883 she sent a wreath of flowers to be laid at its foot. During his visits Goethe wrote a number of odes on subjects connected with Carlsbad.

The period embracing the close of the eighteenth and commencement of the nineteenth century was the "golden age" of Carlsbad. The royal and noble visitors vied with each other in the originality and costliness of their entertainments. Among the most celebrated *fêtes* was the Chinese banquet given in 1786 by the Countess Ozinska, when the Alte Wiese was lighted with 1500 coloured lanterns and lined with small pavilions decorated with mirrors. On the Pupp'sche Allée an immense Chinese pagoda was erected, in which the servants of the Countess, dressed in Chinese costume, served the feast. Another curious entertainment was given in 1797 by the Duke of Saxe-Gotha to the beautiful Duchess Dorothée of Curland (see page 122). In a meadow near the Franzens Brücke hay was being made, and the Duke had invited all the visitors to take a drive along the Eger. While the carriages were passing the field the Duke suggested that his guests should alight and join in the merriment of the haymakers, who were dancing to the music of pipes and fiddles. His proposal was at once adopted, and after the dance was over their host led the guests to an immense hayrick which stood in the meadow, and from which sounds of music were apparently proceeding. On their approach it fell apart, and disclosed a sumptuous banquet spread on a long table, over one end of which a gallery filled with musicians had been erected. Besides these *fêtes*, there were, almost daily, balls, balloon ascents, chess tournaments, where the places of the chessmen were taken by children suitably attired, and concerts in which the most celebrated musicians in Europe took part.

In 1791 the poet Schiller visited Carlsbad with his wife, to whom he had been married the year before. We gather from his letters written during his stay that the time he passed was the happiest period in his life. It was during this visit that Rheinhardt painted the celebrated portrait of the poet. He lodged at the house 'Zum Weissen Schwan,' near the Johannisbrücke.

In 1809 the town suffered severely in the French war, the number of guests being reduced from 1200 the year previous, to 112. In 1813 the visitors from Saxony and Poland and other states then at war with Saxony were ordered to leave the baths within three days. In 1819 the celebrated conference which was held to decide the settlement of Europe after the Napoleonic wars, and which lasted from 7th August to 20th December, assembled at Carlsbad, in the Hotel Zum Weissen Löwen. Shortly after the battle of

Waterloo Marshal Blucher paid a visit to Carlsbad, and was much fêted by the Cur-guests. He is said to have remarked that "he had been an enemy to water all his life, but now the devil had sent him where he could get nothing else."

In 1830 the new bath-houses were commenced, and other improvements in the town and environs were undertaken. In 1852 the present Cur-tax was established, and visitors were no longer received as formerly by a flourish of trumpets from the Stadtthurm. In 1858 the 500th anniversary of the legendary discovery of the baths by the Emperor Charles IV. was held amid great rejoicing.

Besides the distinguished visitors already mentioned Carlsbad has been honoured by visits from Frederick I., 1708, and Frederick William I., of Prussia, 1732; the Emperor Joseph II. of Austria, 1766; the Empress Marie Ludovika, 1810; King Anthony of Saxony, 1812; the Emperor Francis I. and his daughter Maria Louisa, second wife of Napoleon I., 1812; William III., 1816; the Empress Maria Feodorowna of Russia, 1818; King Ernest of Hanover, 1837; King Otho of Greece, 1856; the present German Emperor, 1864; the Crown Prince and Princess of Prussia, 1870; the Emperor and Empress of Brazil, 1872; the ex-Empress of the French, 1883.

Besides these royalties the Cur-books at Carlsbad are inscribed with the names of Bach, Beethoven, Catalani, Sontag, Paganini, Schopenhauer, Wellington, Prince

Metternich, Kroner, Chateaubriand, Auerbach, Tourgenieff, Prince Bismarck, John Bright, and the late Lord Ampthill.

Carlsbad has many times suffered severely from inundations of the Tepel, notably in May 1582, when three-fourths of the houses were swept away and many of the inhabitants drowned; in February 1655, when eighteen houses were destroyed; and in September 1821, when all the bridges and a great part of the wall along the Tepel were carried away, and the goods in the shops on the river-bank were almost entirely destroyed, the water reaching the second floor of the houses. Great destruction has also several times been worked by the breaking out of the Sprudel. On the 22d February 1799, in consequence of the sudden breaking-up of the ice, the spring burst through the ground, carrying everything before it, and then almost disappeared,—in consequence of which a rumour spread that the spring had been swallowed up by an earthquake. This was a serious calamity for Carlsbad, as a total cessation of the drinking of the waters took place in consequence. It was months before the spring was replaced, it being necessary to level the bed of the river and pave the sides with massive slabs of granite, while its banks had to be sealed with cement. In 1604 the town was almost entirely distroyed by fire, only three houses being left standing, and again in 1759, when 224 houses were burned to the ground.

A sketch of the history of Carlsbad would not be

complete without reference being made to its celebrated K. K. Schützen-Corps, or Royal and Imperial Shooting Corps. This society is a very ancient one, having been orginally a company of crossbowmen. The date of the foundation of the society is unknown, but its first royal charter was granted in 1630. One of the ancient privileges of Carlsbad was that no military should be quartered in the town, and there being therefore no garrison, the shooting corps have always undertaken the duties of the town guard. The corps wear a handsome uniform of green and gold, and the visitor to Carlsbad will have many opportunities of seeing them marching through the town headed by their band. The shooting matches of the society have been patronised by most of the royal and noble visitors to Carlsbad since its foundation, who have written their names in the autograph-book, and have presented a number of prizes to be shot for. This book and many of the prizes are preserved in the Schiesshaus in the Schützen Park, and form a most interesting collection. Weekly shooting matches are still held on Sundays, at which visitors are made welcome, and allowed to take part.

IV.

LIFE AT CARLSBAD.

CARLSBAD has now settled down, after the gay days of her *première jeunesse*—when her princely and noble visitors accompanied the drinking of the waters with a continual round of gaiety —to follow again the sound maxim of old Dr. Payer, "that Nature hath created this bath for patients, and not for anybody's lust or amusement." When he reads of the open-air *fêtes*, the balls, and the nightly illuminations given by the distinguished guests, where all were welcome, the visitor of to-day may naturally feel tempted to regret the change in the social life at Carlsbad, when he finds his days bound by rigid rules, and himself but a unit of a crowd of health-seekers who, from their very number and difference of station and nationality, are debarred from that free social intercourse which doubtless most would desire if it were possible.

There are many reasons that account for this change. In earlier days the guests were few in number, and were nearly all of the "upper classes," with some crowned head or star of fashion as their presiding genius. To-

CARLSBAD—STADT PARK.

day this select circle has gradually extended to a mingled concourse, drawn from all countries and classes of the civilised world, with few able to lead, and fewer willing to follow, in any revival of the old festivities. All now must feel themselves more or less strangers in this vast throng, and be content to devote themselves to the business of the hour, and to seek their enjoyment amid their own immediate circle, and in the happy consciousness of returning health. But in spite of the barriers to general intercourse among the visitors, there is withal a kindly tone in the social life at Carlsbad, doubtless owing greatly to the leaven of the geniality of the Austrian character, and there are many quiet and healthful pleasures, particularly suited to those who have come in search of health and repose.

The cure at Carlsbad is by no means a "fancy" cure. It is no place for those who wish to make a visit to a watering-place simply in search of amusement or gaiety. Here there is no extravagance either in the mode of life or in fashionable display. The goddess of health reigns supreme, and all must yield to her sway. But after all he must be a discontented and unappreciative mortal indeed who cannot find amusement enough in the pleasant summer days at Carlsbad, with its charming drives and walks, its promenades and cafés, where he can mingle with the passing throng, or can rest luxuriously beneath some shady chestnut tree, and wile away the hours in friendly intercourse, or in listening to the music of the orchestra; or perchance, if weary, and wishing solitude, he can seek refuge with a favourite author in some sequestered nook,—returning health and the hope of a speedy recovery adding zest to every pleasure.

"Early to bed and early to rise" is the strict rule at Carlsbad, and the visitor must be prepared for the—perhaps at first unwelcome—rap at half-past five; but when once up and dressed, what can be more delightful than the first fresh cool hours of the summer mornings and the first singing of the birds, which are so carefully looked after by the kindly peasantry for the welcome of the guests? At six the visitor seeks the health-restoring springs, and takes his morning goblet from the hands of the neatly dressed little maid who presides over the fountain; and here let us advise him to be early at the well, and so save himself many tedious waits in the slowly advancing line of two or three hundred other patients, which have to be repeated for as many glasses as he is ordered to drink. This trouble can be avoided, however, by hiring a 'dienstmann' (see page 81) for 20 kr., who will stand in the line and hand the cup to the visitor when his turn comes. After drinking, a promenade is taken, enlivened by the strains of the band and the curious sight of a long line of people, of many climes and many costumes, solemnly waiting their turn, cup in hand, at the spring. After each cup another walk is taken, until the prescribed quantity has been taken. Then to breakfast;—and now, to the newly arrived English or American visitor, comes the rub. Accustomed at home to his substantial morning meal, it does seem hard at first, after a good hour's exercise in the fresh morning air, to have to content himself with a cup of coffee and a roll purchased at the nearest bakery. He is not even allowed butter, unless he happens to have an indulgent doctor, who will allow him just enough to remind him of his boarding-school days. But there is no help for it; he has come for the "cure," and must abide by its rules. One solace, however, is left him, few doctors being so hard-hearted as to deny just one pipe or cigar. The rest of the morning is spent at the Curhaus perusing the newspapers, with which the reading rooms are plentifully supplied, or in a short drive or gentle stroll, until the bathing-hour comes round; after which the visitor returns to his hotel refreshed and invigorated with the bracing mineral or luxurious peat bath. The dinner-hour at Carlsbad is primitive, but to the hungry visitor who has gone through a long morning on a roll and a cup of coffee, it is welcome enough. The dinner of the Cur-guest, however, must be simple and in keeping with his Arcadian life; but, with soup, fish, a roast joint, green vegetables, stewed fruit, and the *sauce piquante* of a healthy appetite, he has little ground for complaint. Nor is he obliged to join the Army of the Blue Ribbon; in moderation he can take claret, hock, light German beer, or better still, and most refreshing, the country wines of Bohemia, diluted with sparkling Giesshübl or Krondorfer water. Dinner over, another walk is taken, for even "forty winks," however tempting in the drowsy summer weather, are strictly forbidden. And so passes the day, till the sun begins to drop behind the wooded hills, when all Carlsbad turns out at its gayest to promenade, to see and be seen, or to sit at the little tables under the trees and drink the most aromatic coffee in the world, so cheerfully served by the young and pretty coffee-girls.

At the cafés or in the Curgarten Labitzky's band discourses sweet music from four to six, and on the Alte Wiese and the Pupp'sche Allée there is a constant ebb and flow of promenaders, amongst whom the lively and exquisitely dressed daughters of Austria and Hungary, we must unpatriotically say, bear away the palm for style and beauty. The concert ended, the visitors soon disperse; and a light supper taken, the fine new theatre or the evening concerts at the Curhaus are now the attractions, or if it be a Saturday—the fête-day of the week, on which visitors, like children of a larger growth, are allowed to "stay up"—the ballroom at the Curhaus is opened, and from eight till twelve, to the strains of Labitzky's band, dancing goes on with the full consent of even our tyrant the Cur physician. These are no formal gatherings; the "swallow-tail" of civilisation finds no place in the simple life at Carlsbad, and ladies are expressly requested to appear in "*toilette de ville;*" but, nevertheless, these dances are most enjoyable from their very freedom from restraint and ceremony. On other evenings Carlsbad is in bed by ten, for early to rise means early to rest.

V.

ARRIVAL—HOTELS—LODGINGS—CAFÉS AND BEST SHOPS.

ON crossing the Austrian frontier the luggage of travellers is examined by the Customs; but tobacco and spirits, and uncut pieces of silk or velvet are practically the only articles on which duty is levied. The Custom-House officers are extremely civil, but to avoid all chance of trouble the traveller should declare at once any dutiable articles he may have in his luggage.

Passports are not now required in Austria. It is nevertheless advisable to carry one as a means of personal identification.

On arrival at the station the traveller will find carriages and omnibuses from the hotels in waiting. If he has chosen his hotel he should seek out the hotel porter, who will look after his luggage and see him comfortably settled in his carriage or omnibus. The traveller should try and so arrange his journey as to arrive at Carlsbad early in the evening, when, if he have not secured apartments beforehand, he should proceed to a hotel for the night, and next day look for lodgings at his leisure. The choice of lodgings, however, being a matter of great importance, it is better, in the height of the season, to secure them if possible beforehand. The doctor to whom the visitor is recommended will willingly render all assistance in his power on receiving particulars of the case, the accommodation required, and the expected date of arrival, and his advice as to the most desirable locality suited to the patient will be found most valuable. The prices of rooms, of course, depend very much on the situation and the period of the year at which they are taken. Apartments in the Alte Wiese, Park Strasse, Neue Wiese, or on the heights of the Schlossberg are much dearer than those in the Prager Gasse, the Kreutz Gasse, or the Eger Strasse. Between the 15th May and 15th July the prices are twice as much as during the rest of the year. During the height of the season single bedrooms can be had from 10 to 20 fl. per week, a suite of two to four rooms between 20 and 50 fl. a week, and large suites from 100 to 200 fl. a week.

The hotels in Carlsbad are exceedingly comfortable, and the prices compare favourably with those of other fashionable watering-places. The rooms are generally large, airy, and well furnished, and the cooking is good. The average prices in hotels of the first class are— from April to May, salon and bedroom, 15 to 30 fl. per week; single bedrooms, 8 to 12 fl., and per day about 2 fl. From June to July, salon and bedroom, 30 to 60 fl. per week; single bedroom, 12 to 20 fl., and per day, 3 fls. During August and September the prices are the same as in April and May. The price for rooms include service only. Gaslights and candles are about 25 kr. each, lamps 35 kr. per day, fires 50 kr. per day. The charge for service does not include the porter or boots. Visitors should always make a definite arrangement with the proprietor before taking rooms.

The Carlsbad hotels do not furnish *table d'hôte*, as nearly all the visitors are on a special regimen. The meals taken by visitors generally consist of coffee and bread in the morning, generally taken at a café, dinner in the middle of the day, and a light supper in the evening. The average prices charged for meals at the hotels are about as follows:—Coffee with bread, half portion, 36 kr.; whole portion, 60 kr.; eggs, 6 kr. each. Dinner is charged at a fixed price of about 1 fl. 50 kr. to 4 fl., according to the number of dishes ordered.

Soup, beef or mutton, vegetables, a roast dish, and compôt and pudding, 1 guld. 50 kr.

Same as above, with fish, 2 fl.

With fish, ice, and dessert, 3 fl.

With fish, an additional roast dish, entrée, ice, and dessert, 4 fl.

Supper is order *à la carte*, a portion of fish or meat costing from 50 to 80 kr. One portion, as in France, can be shared by two.

The second-class hotels are generally about 20 per cent. cheaper, although in some cases they are just as dear as the first class, and should vistors intend to stay in any of them a bargain should be made beforehand.

Hotels of the first class are—*Anger's Hotel*, Neue Wiese, adjoining the new theatre; *Pupps' Hotel*, Pupp'sche Allée; *Königs Villa*, Theresien Park; *Goldener Schild*, with *dépendances*, *Erzherzog Stephan* and *Zwei Deutsche Monarchen; Hotel Hanover*, Markt; *Hotel National*, Neue Gartenzeile; *Hotel de Russie*, Kaiserstrasse.

Hotels of the second class are:—*Donau*, Parkstrasse; *Paradies*, Kaiserstrasse; *Drei Fasanen*, Kirchengasse; *Erzherzog Karl*, Kirchengasse.

All the hotels have restaurants attached.

CAFÉS.—*Pupps'*, on the Alte Wiese (page 109), *Café Schönbrunn* (page 123), *Kaiser Park* (page 114), *Sans Souci* (page 111), *Post Hof* (page 113), *Freundschafts-Salle* (page 113), *Café Saxe*, *Café Zum Elephant*, on the Alte Wiese—English and French newspapers; *Café Imperial*, north of the town on the right bank—electric light, concerts.

Coffee at the cafés, 28 kr.; rolls, 2 kr. each. When black coffee is desired the order is given for 'Recht café,' and for weaker coffee, 'Verkehrt.' At all the cafés two cups can be ordered with one portion. If only one cup is wanted, the order is for a 'Kleinen Kapuziner,' for which 16 kr. is charged. The usual custom is to buy the rolls at a baker's, the best being Mannl & Pittroff, in the Alte Wiese, and take them to the café.

The servants at the hotels and lodging-houses, and the attendants at the cafés all expect gratuities. Those given at the hotels and lodgings must of course depend on the length of the visit and the attention shown. At the cafés and restaurants the usual fees are—for coffee, 10 kr.; dinner, 20 kr. to the head waiter, to whom the bill is paid, and 10 kr. to the waiter; supper the same. At the baths the girl who supplies the linen expects about 20 kr., and the male attendant 10 kr. The drivers of the carriages expect a fee of 5 to 10 per cent. on the fare.

Recommendable Shops.

Antiquities and Curiosities—C. J. Meyer, Alte Wiese.
Bohemian Glass—L. Moser, "Rother Adler," Alte Wiese; Holzner, Bahnhof-Str.; A. H. Pfeiffer, 42 Alte Wiese.
Booksellers—Franieck, "Drei Lämmer," Markt; Knauer, Markt; Feller, Markt; Stark, Mühlbadgasse.
Cartridges—Rosenfeld, "Weisser Löwe," Markt.
Chemists—F. Worliczek, Markt, 381; H. R. Lippmann, 17 Mühlbadgasse.
Cigars and Cigarettes—David Moser, Markt; Frank, Sprudelgasse.
Confectioners—W. Stadler, "König von Preussen," Mühlbadgasse; Rumler, Alte Wiese; Bär, Alte Wiese.
Express, Parcels, and Baggage—Ulrich & Gross, Kaiser-Str.; Bartels, Kaiser-Str.

Grocer—Rosenfeld, Sprudelgasse.

Hairdressers and Perfumers—Jelineck & Erdmann, Alte Wiese.

Hatter—Karl Gimm, Mühlbadgasse.

Medical Instruments and Bandages—W. Rusy, Alte Wiese; Berry, Neue Wiese.

Milliners—E. Hein, "Mozart," Alte Wiese; Brüder Nastopil. Alte Wiese, 335.

Opticians—Brüder Teiner, "Goldener Harfe," Alte Wiese.

Photographers—Jerie, Am Quai; Hirsch, Garten Zeil; Wagner, Marienbad-Str.

Pianos (also for hire)—Anton Wiesinger, Hotel National.

Shoemaker—Mannl-Hein, "Goldener Schlüssel," Mühlbadgasse.

Sprudelstein Articles—J. Sebert, Alte Wiese; Tschammerhöll, Sprudel Colonnade.

Tailors—E. Epstein, "Drei Lämmer," Markt; Max Epstein, Wittwe, Markt.

Bankers—

Gottlieb Lederer, Markt; Brüder Benedict, Alte Wiese and Mühlbadgasse; A. Schwalb, Markt; Böhmirche Escompte, Bank Filiall, Mühlbadgasse.

VI.

CONCERTS, THEATRES, AND AMUSEMENTS.

CARLSBAD has a fine theatre, opened 1886 (see p. 90), in which excellent performances of German, French, and Italian plays and operas are given. The box-office is open from 9 till 12. Doors open at 6 P.M.; performance commences at 7.

THEATRE PRICES.

1. *In the Parterre.*

	fl.	kr.
Proscenium boxes for six persons	12	0
Parterre boxes for four persons	7	0
Parquet seats (stalls), first three rows	2	0
,, ,, fourth to eighth rows	1	50
Balcony stalls, first row	2	0
,, ,, second row	1	50
,, ,, third and fourth rows	1	20
First floor boxes—mittelfremdenloge		
First row, four fauteuils	2	20
Second row, four fauteuils	1	60
First row boxes, for five persons	8	0

2. *In the Balcony.*

	fl.	kr.
Middle balcony seat, first row	1	20
,, ,, second to sixth rows	1	0
Side balcony seats, first row	1	10
,, ,, second and third rows	0	70
Amphitheatre	0	50
,, area	0	20

CONCERTS.—From 1st May to 30th September in the Curhaus, on Monday, Wednesday, and Friday, in unfavourable weather from 7.30 to 9 P.M. When the weather is fine the band plays on these evenings—Monday, at the *Café Sans-Souci;* Wednesday, at the *Salle de Saxe;* Friday, in the *Stadtpark;* also in the *Stadtpark*, Sundays from 4 to 6 P.M.; in the garden of the *Café Pupp*, Tuesdays and Thursdays, from 4 to 6 P.M.; and in rainy weather in the salon of the café. The orchestra plays during the drinking hours from 6 to 8 A.M. in the morning daily in the *Sprudel* and *Mühlbrunn* Colonnades. Military and classical concerts are also given in the Cafés *Posthof, Schönbrunn, Sans-Souci*, and *Salle de Saxe*—admission, 50 krs. From the 1st October to 30th April concerts are given in the Curhaus on Tuesday, Friday, and Thursday evenings from 7 to 8.30 P.M., and every alternate Sunday, from 4 to 6 P.M. in the afternoon. The days given above for concerts are liable to alteration.

BALLS are given every Saturday evening at the Curhaus from 8 to 12 P.M.; admission, 1 fl. 50 kr. The finest ball of the year is held on the 18th of August, in honour of the birthday of the Austrian Emperor.

In the SUMMER THEATRE performances of comedy, vaudeville, farce, &c., are given in the afternoon from four to six.

During the season numerous strolling companies of actors, gymnasts, musicians, conjurors, &c., visit Carlsbad.

For shooting and fishing see p. 163.

VII.

TOWN REGULATIONS.

Cure and Music Tax.

ALL visitors to Carlsbad who remain over eight days, whether taking the cure or not, are subject to the cure and music taxes, which are divided into four classes.

Cure-Tax.

1st Class.—Which embraces noblemen, officers, Government employees, the superior priesthood, land-owners, independent gentry, professional men, merchants, bankers, manufacturers, and well-to-do people generally . . . . 10 fl.

2d Class.—People of moderate means . 6 „

3d Class.—The working classes, small shop-keepers, and people of small means . . 4 „

4th Class.—Children under fourteen and servants . . . . 1 „

Doctors and surgeons, military officers under the rank of captain, and their wives, widows and children, are exempt from the cure-tax, but pay a reduced music-tax.

Music-Tax.

				fl.
1st Class.—One person				5
,,	A party of 2 persons			8
,,	,,	3 ,,		11
,,	,,	4 ,,		14
,,	,,	5 ,,	or more	17
2d Class.—One person				3
,,	A party of 2 persons			5
,,	,,	3 ,,		6
,,	,,	4 ,,		7
,,	,,	5 ,,	or more	8
3d Class.—One person				2
,,	A party of 2 persons			3
,,	,,	3 ,,		4
,,	,,	4 ,,		5
,,	,,	5 ,,	or more	6

Children under fourteen and servants pay no music-tax.

The " cure-tax " does not include admission to the reading and smoking rooms. Tickets for these rooms can be purchased at the office. Daily tickets, 15 kr.; weekly, 70 kr.; monthly, 2 fl.

The taxes are assessed by the Burgomaster, but any visitor objecting to his assessment can appeal against it within three days, by lodging a notice in writing at either the office of the Burgomaster, in the Town Hall, or at the office of the District Surveyor in the Municipal Buildings on the Neue Wiese. Shortly after his arrival each visitor is supplied with a form of assessment to fill up, which is returned a few days afterwards for payment. A List of Regulations is issued annually by the Burgomaster and circulated among the visitors.

REGULATIONS RESPECTING LODGINGS.

1. Any stranger arriving in Carlsbad is permitted to hire a lodging either for a fixed or for an indefinite period of time. With respect to rent, and all other arrangements entered into, written or verbal contracts are considered equally binding. To save disputes, however, it is better to have a contract in writing. (See Rule 13.)

2. If the lodging is hired for a fixed period, the contract made is considered in force during the whole of the time the rooms are occupied; and when the period originally fixed on has expired, and the stay is prolonged, no further contract is necessary, unless an alteration in the terms be agreed on, in which case a new contract must be made.

3. The fact of the rent being paid weekly (as is usual) has no bearing upon the contract, *i.e.*, a week's notice on either side is not sufficient when the apartments have been hired by the month.

4. During the continuance of a contract for a fixed period, the owner of the lodgings cannot increase the rent.

5. If the lodgings be rented for an indefinite

period, and no special contract have been made, it is assumed that the visitor has hired the apartments for the usual time of taking the waters, viz., four weeks; but during this time the landlord cannot insist on any increase in the rent originally agreed on. In this case, if the hirer wishes to vacate the apartments at the end of the fourth week, or if the landlord wishes to let them to some other person, a week's notice beforehand is necessary. Should this not be given, the contract runs on for an indefinite period, and can be put an end to at any time by either party giving a week's notice.

6. If apartments are expressly rented by the day, it is only necessary to give a notice of twenty-four hours on either side; or, if by the week, a week's notice.

7. The week's notice is reckoned from the day on which the weekly payment becomes due. If notice be given during the course of the week, it is only regarded as having been given at the expiration of the week.

8. If, in the case of a lodging which is hired either by the week or for an indefinite period, the lodger gives notice to leave at any time during the first day he takes possession, he cannot be required to pay more than the rent for the current week.

9. If the visitor who has hired his apartments either by the week or for an indefinite period desires to quit his lodgings suddenly, he has not only to pay the rent for the current week, but also the amount of an additional week's rent as compensation in lieu of

E

notice; but at the same time, he cannot sublet the apartments for this unexpired period to any other person. In the case of lodgings being hired by the day, the compensation in lieu of notice is one day's rent.

10. All persons letting lodgings have a right to demand a deposit from the hirer, which, however, must not exceed the amount of one week's rent. The deposit is forfeited if the hirer shall not take possession of the lodging during the course of the first week. This rule does not apply if the hirer furnishes the owner with sufficient security for his fulfilling the terms of his contract. Should such security not be furnished, the landlord has the right, at the termination of the week, to cancel the contract and let the lodgings to any other person.

11. In hotels and boarding-houses, visitors have the right to vacate their apartments at any time they please, and only to pay by the day. Should, however, a visitor hire apartments in a hotel or boarding-house for a fixed price, and for a period longer than one day (whether it be for a fixed or indefinite period), the above regulations applicable to lodging-houses come into force.

12. If the stipulations of the contract are not kept by the landlord—that is, if the visitor shall not be provided with that which is contracted for, or what may be said to come under the head of necessities; if it can be proved that the lodging is damp, dirty, or in any way injurious to health; or if facts come to light which the hirer had no means of discovering at the

time of his entering into the contract, whereby he may be inconvenienced; and provided such causes of complaint are not immediately removed by the landlord, the lodger shall have the right of vacating the apartments without notice; but he must pay for the actual time he has occupied the apartments.

13. In such cases the onus of proof lies upon the lodger; and also if any dispute arises as to whether the lodging was hired for a fixed or an indefinite period, the onus of proof lies with the person who raises the dispute. If no written contract has been made between the parties, and a dispute takes place regarding a verbal contract, the arrival-sheet, which contains a column stating the period for which the visitor proposes to stay, shall be taken as proof. In cases where this is not recorded in the arrival-sheet, the assertion of the visitor is taken as proof.

14. In the case of furnished lodgings, no compensation can be claimed for injury or deterioration sustained by the furniture, linen, &c., by ordinary wear and tear, but compensation can be claimed where anything has been wilfully broken or damaged, and in cases of severe or prolonged illness, where any large amount of bed-linen is required, or when from this cause any articles have been rendered unfit for further use.

15. Every visitor has the right to procure his meals, food, and necessaries, as well as to take his baths, where he pleases. He has also the right of having his own laundress.

16. The rent does not usually include attendance, unless it has been expressly stipulated in the contract. Where no arrangement shall have been made for attendance, it shall be determined according to the tariff usual in the house. When attendance is charged in the usual monthly or weekly account, and shall have been thus paid to the landlord by the lodger, the servants have no claim to separate gratuities.

The term "attendance" is understood to mean usual domestic services, such as the cleaning and putting in order of the rooms, attending at meals, and other services usually rendered by domestics; but ironing of linen, washing, mending, and cleaning of clothes and boots, or attending upon the sick are expressly excluded.

17. All disputes arising between visitors and lodging-house keepers must be laid before the Royal District Assessor, at the Amtsgebäude, or district offices, Neue Wiese, who will use his best endeavours to arrange the matters in dispute satisfactorily; but, failing this, he shall then direct the parties to apply to the law courts. When, however, both parties shall agree that the District Assessor shall be called upon to arbitrate the matter, his decision shall be final.

Bath Regulations.

1. The public baths of the town are under the direct control of the municipality of Carlsbad, subject to the general supervision of the Government.

2. When baths are ordered, they will be allotted by the cashier according to priority of application.

3. The baths are open to the public from morning till evening.

4. Tickets for a bath, or for a series of baths, are issued in the establishment by the cashier or the bath attendants at the prices fixed by the tariff. Only tickets obtained in this way are available. The tickets must be paid for in advance.

5. The ticket is only available at the establishment where it is bought and for the hour arranged.

6. In case the patient cannot take the bath at the hour arranged for, at least two hours' notice must be given in advance, otherwise the price of the ticket will not be refunded.

7. The ticket must be delivered to the attendant on entering the bath-room.

8. Bathers must be punctual to the hours mentioned on the ticket, the time allowed being one hour for each bath. A bell is rung fifteen minutes before the expiration of the hour to give the bather warning to dress and vacate the bath-room.

9. Every bather has the right to request that his bath shall be prepared in his presence; and in order to assure himself that the temperature of the bath is exactly that desired, a thermometer is placed in each bath-room.

10. The bath attendants must obey strictly all orders

given for the preparation of the baths, and must treat bathers with proper civility.

11. The bath attendants are strictly enjoined to keep the bath-rooms clean and in order; and bathers are also urgently requested not to damage or soil the bath-rooms in any way.

12. Smoking and the use of strong smelling liniments are strictly forbidden.

13. A bell will be found in each cabinet, which can be rung in case of necessity.

14. The bath inspectors and attendants are strictly forbidden to interfere with the comfort of the bathers.

15. Any disorder in the bath-rooms, negligence, or incivility on the part of the bath attendants, or other cause of complaint, must be written in the complaint book, which will be found in the waiting-room, and which duly comes under the notice of the municipality.

16. It is strictly forbidden to bring dogs into the Curhaus or bath-rooms.

17. The use of the common baths is given free to the poor, who, however, must produce a legal certificate of their inability to pay.

Bath Tariff.

	fl.	kr.
One mineral salon bath in the Curhaus, morning or evening, with service	1	50
One mineral bath in the Curhaus or in the other bath-houses, after 2 P.M., with service	1	0
One mineral bath in do. before 2 P.M., with service	0	70

	fl.	kr.
One mineral douche bath, with service	1	50
One Russian steam bath and cold douche, without service	1	0
One cold douche bath, without service	0	60
One peat bath, including a bath of fresh water afterwards, as follows:—		
With 48 kilogrammes of peat	2	0
„ 60 „ „	2	30
„ 72 „ „	2	60
„ 84 „ „	2	80
„ 96 „ „	3	0
One salon peat bath in the new Curhaus bath	3	0
One iron bath	1	0
One bath at the Sauerbrunnen	1	0
One fresh-water bath, with service	1	0
Each person in the public bath	0	5
Heating the bath-room with woodfire	0	20

Use of Bath Linen.

	fl.	kr.
Each bath-gown	0	20
Each bath-sheet	0	10
Each towel	0	4

Where a salon bath is taken, the price of bath linen is double these rates.

In the Curhaus only peat baths can be had.

	fl.	kr.
With 6 kilogrammes of earth	0	24
„ 12 „ „	0	48
Bran in addition, each 3 kilos.	0	50

	fl.	kr.
Carlsbad Sprudel soap-lye, per litre . . .	0	20
Carlsbad Sprudel-lye salt, per kilo. . . .	1	0
With Sprudel soap in addition	0	70
Sea-salt, 2 to 5 kilos., per kilo. . . .	0	40
Common-salt, 2 to 5 kilos., per kilo. . .	0	20

In every bath-house there is a complaint book.

REGULATIONS FOR PUBLIC CARRIAGES.

1. The hirer is at liberty to select any vehicle he may choose, without regard to its position upon the rank.

2. Where the carriage is hired by the hour, the fare commences from the time of engaging the carriage. Where the fare is paid by distance, a delay of ten minutes is allowed; beyond this time, for each half-hour's waiting, for a one-horse carriage, 40 kr.; two-horse carriage, 60 kr. For a longer time, in which a wait of three hours is included, for each half-hour's delay beyond this time, one-horse carriage, 20 kr.; two-horse carriage, 30 kr.

3. From 9 P.M. to 6 A.M. half-fare additional is charged. If the carriage is hired by the hour, during the day, and is kept beyond 9 P.M., half-fare additional is to be paid for the time after that hour.

4. No charge is made for small articles taken inside the carriage. For luggage carried outside a one-horse carriage, not exceeding 1½ cwt., 30 kr., and on a two-horse carriage, not exceeding 2 cwt., 50 kr.

5. Should the carriage, after being hired, be countermanded by the hirer, a compensation of one florin for a one-horse carriage, and 1 fl. 50 krs. for a two-horse carriage must be paid, unless the delay, if reckoned by time, entitle the driver to more.

6. The driver of a carriage can in no case decline to take a fare, unless he can show it to be impossible to undertake it.

7. If the drive be interrupted by any accident to either the driver or his vehicle, he has no claim whatever on the hirer.

8. If the driver of a public vehicle have accepted an engagement, he shall make it known by laying his whip down on his seat.

9. The driver is bound to supply the hirer with the same carriage as he had in use when hired; and, unless by the express consent of the hirer, he cannot transfer the contract to any other driver.

10. Public carriages are required, when conveying a fare, to proceed at a trot whenever the ground will permit.

11. The driver is bound, whenever he is hired by time, to show the hirer his watch and to call attention to it; should he fail to do this, the time, as computed by the hirer, will be assumed to be correct without further question.

12. One-horse carriages are bound to be capable of holding three persons, and two-horse carriages five persons.

13. The driver is not permitted, unless with the express consent of the hirer, to convey any other person either in the carriage or on the box.

14. Each carriage is bound to have hung in the carriage a *fahr-billeten* block; on the front of the leaves of this block a tariff of fares must be printed. The back of the leaf may be used by the passenger for making any complaint, which should be sent to the Burgomaster at Carlsbad, either by being at once handed to a policeman or sent through the post.

Fares.

Fares to any place not mentioned in this list are left to be a matter of private arrangement between the driver and hirer.

By Time.

I. For driving within the precincts of Carlsbad (bounded by the Egerbrücke, Salzsudhaus, Bürgerversorgungshaus, along the main road to the Reichsadler, Helenenhof, Bellaria, English Church, and by the Parkstrasse and the Alte Bahnhofstrasse)—

	fl.	kr.
Two-horse carriage for the first $\frac{1}{2}$ hour	1	20
,, ,, ,, every subsequent $\frac{1}{2}$ hour	0	60
One-horse carriage for the first $\frac{1}{4}$ hour	0	50
,, ,, ,, beyond $\frac{1}{4}$ and less than $\frac{1}{2}$ hour	0	80
,, ,, ,, for every subsequent $\frac{1}{4}$ hour	0	20

TOWN REGULATIONS.

By Distance.	Two-horse Carriage.		One-horse Carriage.	
	fl.	kr.	fl.	kr.
II. From any point within the precincts of the town for the drive—				
To Sans-Souci (Karlsbrücke) Schönbrunn, Posthof, Hospital, Swimmingbath, Klein-Versailles	1	0	0	70
To Jägerhaus, Donitzer Waterworks, Drahowitz, Cemetery, Freundschaftssaal, Kaiserpark	1	50	1	0
To Restaurant Leibold at Pirkenhammer	2	50	1	50
To Aberg, Leonhard, Bergwirthshaus, Zettlitz, Schwarzenbergbrücke, Aich, Dallwitz, Fischern, Pirkenhammer (including the factories)	3	0	2	0
III. From any point within the precincts of the town, including a stay of three hours and return drive—				
To Altrohlau	6	0	4	0
To Schlackenwerth, Lichtenstadt, Tüppelsgrün, Engelhaus	6	70	4	50
To Elbogen, Giesshübl-Puchstein, Giesshübler Porcelain Works	8	0	5	0
To Petschau, Buchau	9	0	6	0
To Joachimsthal	10	0	7	0
To Hauenstein, Welchau	12	0	8	0
To Schlackenwerth and back through Lichtenstadt				
Through Fischern, Altrohlau, Tüppelsgrün and Edersgrün to Lichtenstadt and back				
To Elbogen and back through Schlaggenwald and Pirkenhammer	9	0	6	0
To Elbogen, fetching the passengers from Hans Heilings Warteplatz and back through Aich or Hammer				
To Giesshübl-Puchstein and back along the Schlackenwerther Chaussee				
To Giesshübl and back along the Schlackenwerther Chaussee but allowing time to see Schlackenwerth	10	0	7	0

IV. From the *Railway Station*.
 1. To any point within the town or *vice versâ*—

	fl.	kr.
Two-horse carriage	2	0
One-horse ,,	1	20

 2. To any of the places mentioned above in §§ II. or III. or *vice versâ*—
  (*a*) For all places on the right bank of the Eger, in addition to the regular fare as above mentioned—

Two-horse carriage	1	20
One-horse ,,	0	60

  (*b*) For all places on the left bank of Eger, deduct from the regular fare as above mentioned—

Two-horse carriage	1	20
One-horse ,,	0	60

Stands.

For two-horse vehicles: Theaterplatz and Kaiserstrasse.
For one-horse vehicles: Marktplatz, Geweihdiggasse, Sprudelgasse, Lower Kaiserstrasse and Parkstrasse, behind the military baths.

Regulations for Hiring Donkeys and Donkey-Carriages.

The office where orders are taken is in the Stadthaus, in the Mühlbadgasse (first floor, Stadtkassa).

Fares.

	fl.	kr.
For the whole day	4	50
For the whole day, if hired for one week or more	4	0
For half a day	3	0
During the forenoon: for a ride or drive to the Kreuzberg, the Hirschensprung, or any other place at a similar distance . .	1	50
During the forenoon: for a ride or drive, on level ground, per hour	0	80
Drive to the springs or baths within the town, including the Eisen- and Sauerbrunn baths, with or without return drive	0	80

The drivers are not entitled to ask for any douceur, as they are employed by the town.

For any ride or drive commenced in the forenoon, but not completed until after 1 P.M., the fare for the day has to be paid.

The fares for conveyance to the baths are only in force until 1 o'clock P.M.; after which time half a day must be paid for.

If any other object than a mere visit to the baths be combined with a ride or drive thither, the fare according to time comes at once into force.

In ordering donkeys the following regulations must be observed:—

Only such orders as are lodged at the above office will be attended to.

Owing to the distance of the stables from the office, it is requested that orders may be given at least half an hour before the animal is required.

More than one grown-up person or two children under the age of twelve years are not allowed to sit in the carriage. A contravention of this rule will involve the driver in punishment. He is also not permitted to make his donkey go faster than a walking pace.

Payment must be made in advance, and the hirer will be provided with a ticket, which is only available on the day of issue. Afternoon excursions can only be countermanded up to 12 o'clock noon.

It is requested that any improper behaviour on the part of the driver may be at once reported to the town officials in the above-named office.

Omnibuses.

To the station from the Becher Platz, opposite the Hotel Goldener Schild, every hour before the departure of the trains. Fare, 40 kr.; each piece of luggage, 10 kr.

To *Leibold's Restaurant* and *Pirkenhammer* from the Theater Platz, Neuewiese, 1st May to 30th September:—

From Carlsbad Theater-Platz:	Arrive at Leibold's Restaurant:	Arrive at Pirkenhammer:
1.30 P.M.	2 P.M.	2.10 P.M.
2 ,,	2.30 ,,	2.40 ,,
3 ,,	3.30 ,,	3.40 ,,
3.30 ,,	4 ,,	4.10 ,,

TOWN REGULATIONS.

Return from	
Pirkenhammer to the Leibold Restaurant. :	Leibold Restaurant to Carlsbad :
2.10 P.M.	5.30 P.M.
2.40 ,,	6 ,,
3.40 ,,	6.30 ,,
4.10 ,,	7 ,,
5.10 ,,	...

Fare, 40 kr.

Omnibuses also run to *Erb's Restaurant, Habsburg,* and *Pirkenhammer,* starting from the Goldener Thurm, Sprudelgasse—

Leaving Carlsbad at 9.30 A.M. and 1.30 and 3 P.M.

Returning at 12.15, 2.15, 4.30, and 6 P.M.

Single fare, 40 kr.

To *Aich,* from 1st May to 30th September, from the Theatre Platz—

Leaving Carlsbad at 1.30 and 3.30 P.M.

Returning at 5.30 and 7 P.M.

Single fare, 40 kr.

To *Dallwitz,* from 1st May to 30th September, from the Dienstmann Institut, on the Becher Platz—

Leaving Carlsbad at 1.30 and 3.30 P.M.

Returning at 5 and 7 P.M.

Single fare, 60 kr.   Return fare, 1 fl.

To *Giesshübl Puchstein,* from 1st May to 30th September, starting from the omnibus office on the Becher Platz—

Leaving Carlsbad at 11 A.M. and 1 P.M.

Returning at 6 P.M.

Return fare, 1 fl. 50 kr.

To *Petschau*, from the Post-Office, 12.30 P.M.; return, 6.30 P.M. Fare, 1 florin.

To *Neudeck*, from the Post-Office, 6.30 and 11.30 A.M.; return, 6 A.M. and 3 P.M. Two hours. Fare, 90 kreutzers.

POST AND TELEGRAPH REGULATIONS.

The Post and Telegraph Office is in the Markt Platz, and is open in summer 6 A.M. to 12 P.M. (1st May to 30th September), and in winter from 8 A.M. to 9 P.M. For sale of stamps, issuing of post-office orders, and registering of letters, from 7 A.M. to 7 P.M.

There are also branch and pillar post-offices in various parts of the town.

Postal Rates.

Countries.	Prepaid, each 15 grammes (½ oz.)	Post-cards, each 2 grammes.	Printed matter, prepaid, each 50 grammes (1¾ oz.)
Austria, Germany	5 kr.	2 kr.	2 kr.
Montenegro and Servia	7 „	4 „	2 „
All other European countries, Canada and the United States of America	10 „	5 „	3 „
South America and Asia	20 „	8 „	6 „

Unstamped letters are forwarded, but double postage is collected on delivery. Only Austrian post-cards and stamps are available.

Telegraph Rates.

Austria-Hungary—
  A first charge of 24 kr., and each word . 2 kr.
France—
  First 5 words 60 kr., and each additional word . . . . 12 ,,
Great Britain and Ireland—
  First 5 words 85 kr., and for each additional word . . . . . . 17 ,,
German Empire—
  A first charge of 24 kr., and each word . 6 ,,
Italy—
  A first charge of 24 kr., and each word . 8 ,,
Switzerland—
  Per word . . . . . . 6 ,,
United States and Canada—
  From 1 fl. 27 kr. to 2 fl. 47 kr., according to destination.

In all cases the address and signature must be paid for.

Tariff of the Dienstmann-Institute.
Proprietor—William Knoll.

1. For messages and light employments, or carrying packages up to 15 kilogrammes, ¼ hour, 15 kr.; ½ hour, 20 kr.; 1 hour, 30 kr.; each additional hour, 15 kr.

2. For heavy work, and for messages beyond town limits, ¼ hour, 20 kr.; ½ hour, 30 kr.; 1 hour, 40 kr.; each additional hour, 20 kr.

3. Carrying packages to and from the railway station, 50 to 60 kilogrammes, 60 kr. Each additional 10 kilogrammes, 10 kr.

4. Messages from 9 P.M. to 6 A.M. are charged half as much again as ordinary messages.

Cleaning clothing and boots, per week, each person, 1 florin.

Carrying a piano one way, 2 florins.
,, ,, both ways, 3 florins.

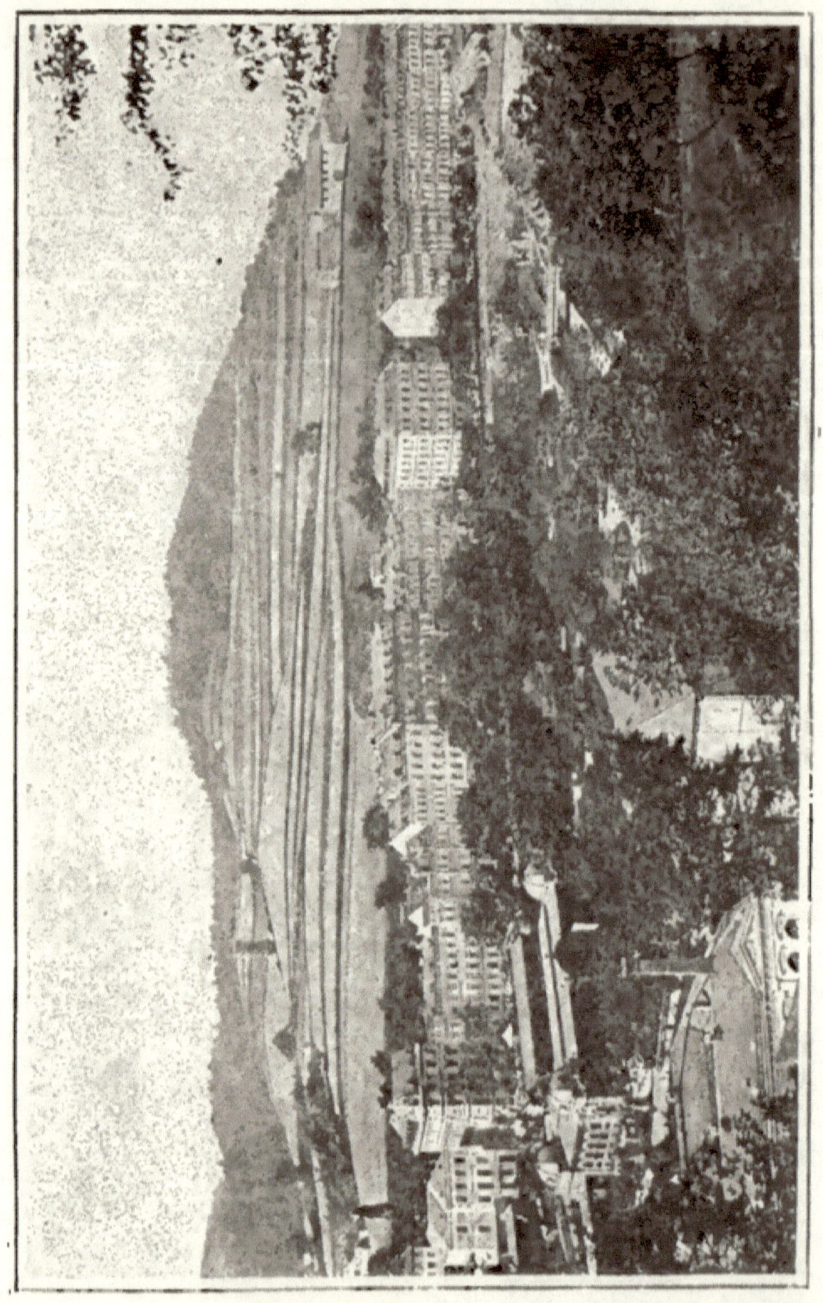
CARLSBAD—GARTENZEILE.

VIII.

DESCRIPTION OF THE TOWN AND PRINCIPAL BUILDINGS.

THE town of Carlsbad consists principally of two long streets, which extend for about a mile on either side of the river Tepel, a clear and rapid stream, which winds through the town in the shape of the letter S, and which is crossed by one large stone, and a number of small iron and wooden bridges. These streets, as we approach from the station, take the names, on the left bank, of the Gartenzeile, Mühlbadgasse, and Alte Wiese; and on the right the Eger Strasse, Kaiser Strasse, Kreuzgasse, Sprudelgasse, and Neue Wiese, the latter being simply portions of the long Marienbad road, which runs through the town. In the centre of the town, on the left bank, is the Markt Platz, in the immediate neighbourhood of which are the Sprudel Colonnade, Mühlbrunn Colonnade, and the Curhaus— the principal places of resort of the visitors. From the Markt Platz along the left bank of the river runs the Alte Wiese, a favourite promenade (see page 109).

The oldest portion of the town is that surrounding the Markt Platz and Sprudel Colonnade, while the newer hotels and villas extend on either side of the Tepel, and line the heights above the left bank. Beyond the Alte Wiese the valley of the Tepel is laid out with beautiful walks and drives, having all the advantages of a large and well-kept park. (For detailed descriptions of the walks and drives see page 109.)

The town at present has about 12,000 inhabitants and 900 houses, mostly hotels and lodging-houses, the majority of which have been built within the last thirty years. At the time of the visit of Charles IV. in 1358, the town only contained forty houses; and even two hundred years later, only consisted of the Markt Platz and the Sprudelgasse. The next streets built were the Kreuzgasse and the Andreasgasse. The first houses on the Alte Wiese were built in 1690, and in 1796 the first shops on the Alte Wiese were erected by the town guilds, in whose possession they remained until 1842, when they were sold to private individuals and rebuilt. None of the buildings in Carlsbad have in themselves any particular historical or architectural interest; but, taken as a whole, the town is well built, and, aided by its natural attractions, it is picturesque and cheerful.

The chief occupation of the inhabitants of Carlsbad is housing, feeding, and generally supplying the wants of its numerous visitors. Its principal industries are the polishing and carving of objects made of sprudel-

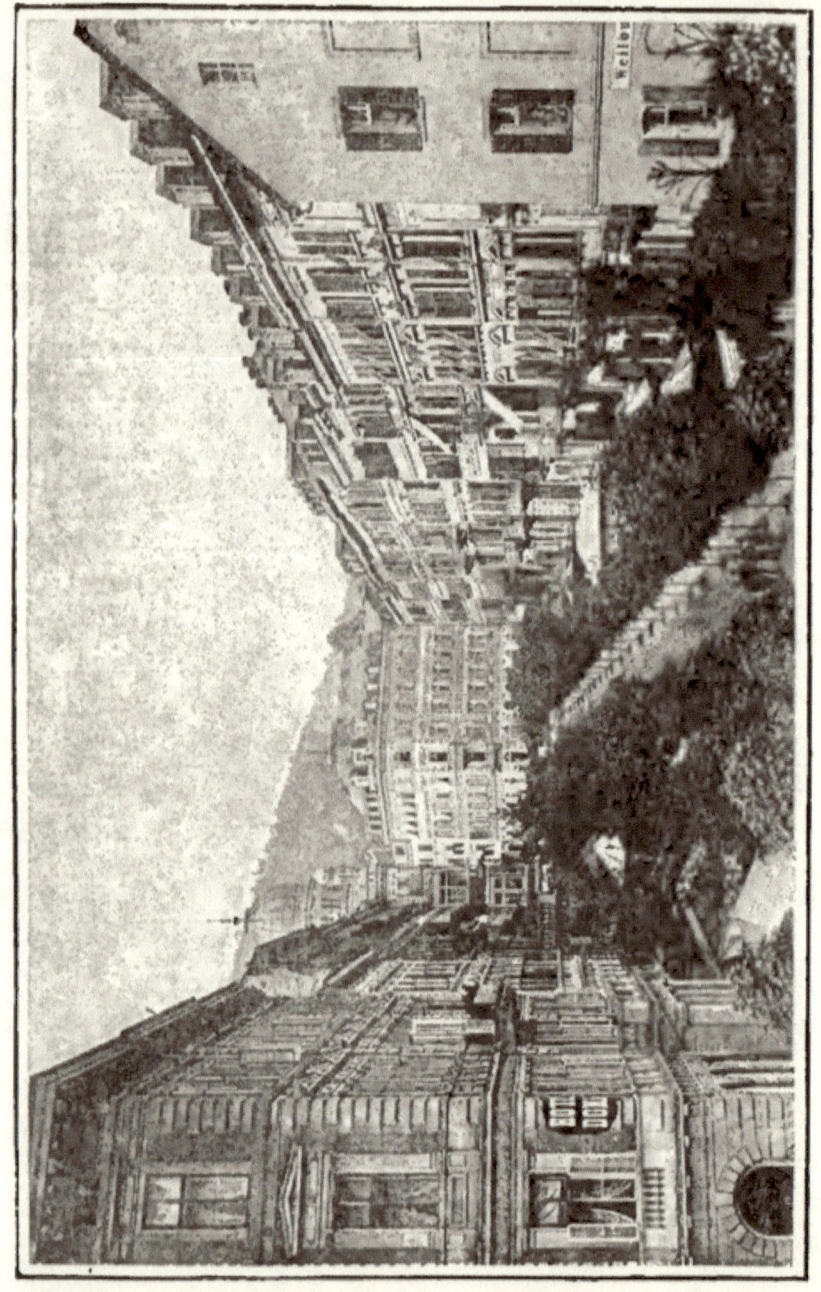

PARKSTRASSE.

stone, the manufacture of the various products of the Carlsbad salts, and of hand-made needles and pins, which latter have quite a celebrity, and which as late as the commencement of this century were known throughout Germany and Austria as "Carlsbad wares." Goethe during one of his visits sent a parcel of Carlsbad pins to his favourite Fraulein von Stein, with a letter telling her they cost 7 marks, "as brass was so dear." There are also a few manufactories of boots and gloves, which are of excellent quality. A considerable trade is carried on in porcelain, which is made in the vicinity.

Other specialties of Carlsbad are "Carlsbad plums," which are prepared by the fruit being partially dried in the sun, and which are even superior to the finest French plums; and "Carlsbad wafers," a thin dessert biscuit, which can be had best at Barbara Bayr's, Königshof.

The inhabitants of Carlsbad are a kindly, intelligent, and industrious people, and always willing to do all in their power to add to the comfort and enjoyment of visitors. An exceedingly pleasant trait in their character is their kindness to birds, of which there are a great number and variety in and around Carlsbad. Killing, and robbing the nests of small birds is strictly forbidden by law, and besides this, a society cares for and feeds them during the winter. The birds are therefore naturally very tame, and any visitor who has a few crumbs to scatter can soon attract numbers of them round him.

The majority of the inhabitants are Roman Catholics, but there are German and English Protestant and Russian churches, as well as a Jewish synagogue.

Public Buildings.

The principal centre of attraction is the *Sprudel Colonnade*, a large and handsome pavilion of iron and glass, erected in 1879 over the Sprudel and Hygeia springs at a cost of 254,000 florins. The principal entrances are from the Sprudelgasse and at the west end. The springs are in the north-east portion of the building, while the south-west portion consists of a large promenade hall, in which is ample space for a thousand people. Here the orchestra plays every morning from six until eight. After drinking each glass of the waters, visitors promenade round the hall to the strains of the band for a quarter of an hour, all being done with the greatest regularity, notices being put up at either end requesting the visitors to circulate from right to left. This long line of promenaders, of many nationalities, with their varied costumes, is one of the most picturesque sights in Europe, to which a grotesque element is lent by the earthenware mugs which each patient carries, either in their hand or, more generally, suspended from their necks. The hall is prettily decorated with palms and flowering plants, while round the walls and up the centre are ranged comfortable seats for the use of the Curguest's spectators. On dark days the hall is brilliantly illuminated by handsome chandeliers. Opposite the orchestra is a monument erected in honour of the celebrated Carlsbad physician, Dr. Becher, died 1792 (see p. 40). Entered from the promenade hall are the rooms containing the springs, which are conducted from the main reservoir by pipes. (For description of the springs see p. 93.)

Beside the Sprudel Colonnade is the *Sprudel Bathhouse*, which contains thirty-six baths; the baths on the ground floor being of porcelain, and on the second floor of metal.

On the opposite side of the river, below the Markt Platz, fronting on the Mühlbrunngasse, is the *Mühlbrunn Colonnade*, a handsome covered promenade of Corinthian architecture, 410 feet in length, supported by 96 pillars, and decorated with eight classical stone statues. The building was completed in 1880 at a cost of 800,000 florins. Under the Colonnade are the Mühlbrunnen (p. 101), Neubrunnen (p. 101), Theresienbrunnen (p. 102), Bernhardsbrunnen (p. 102), and Elizabethquelle (p. 103).

Near the Mühlbrunn Colonnade, and attached to the Stadthaus, is the *Mühlbad*, which is supplied by the waters of the springs in the Mühlbrunn Colonnade. These bath-rooms are exceedingly comfortable and well fitted up, the baths being of porcelain.

The *Stadthaus* is a plain building, erected in 1874 on the foundations of an older structure built in 1510.

Beyond the Muhlbrunn Colonnade is the *Curhaus*, a

large castellated building of little architectural pretensions, erected in 1874–77, at a cost of 350,000 florins. The interior, however, is comfortable, and admirably fitted for the purpose for which it was designed. The lower storey is used for bathing purposes—the bathing rooms being high and well ventilated, and some of them, called "Salon-bäder," are luxuriously fitted up. In all, there are seventy-five mineral baths, twenty-six peat baths, and a Russian steam bath, which, however, is fitted up in a rather primitive style. On this floor there is also a reception room. In the upper storey is a large concert salon, in which concerts and balls are given (p. 61), a restaurant, and three reading-rooms, which are liberally supplied with the principal European newspapers. The English and American newspapers taken are—*The Times, The Daily News, Daily Telegraph, Standard, Illustrated London News, Punch, Galignani's Messenger, New York Herald, Tribune,* and the *American Register.* Readers pay a small fee for admission (see page 63).

To the east of the Curhaus is the *Stranger's Hospital* for poor patients visiting Carlsbad, containing four bed and four bath-rooms. Beyond the Curhaus, to the west, is the *Military Hospital*, in which accommodation is provided for 33 officers and 210 privates. The hospital was built in 1856 from the proceeds of a lottery. In the dining-hall is a large oil-painting by Randler, representing the discovery of the springs at Carlsbad by Charles IV. Admission to the hospital can only be had by an order from the

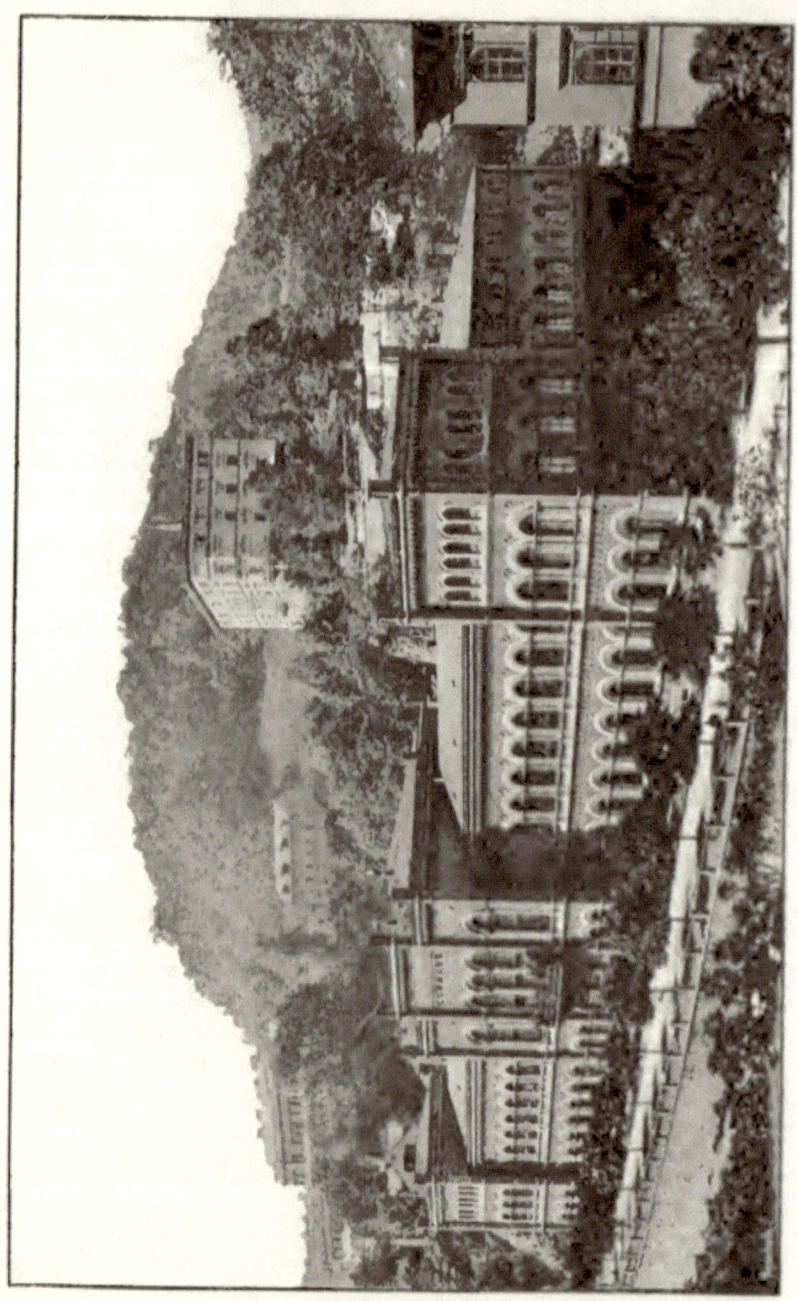

Commandant. The springs which supply the hospital are the Hochbergerquelle and the Kaiserbrunn.

Beyond the hospital is the *Stadt-Park*, a prettily laid out open space, shaded with trees, under which tables and chairs are placed for visitors to drink their coffee, and sit and listen to the band. In the park is an excellent restaurant, open 1st May to 1st September.

On the opposite side of the river, near the stone bridge, is the *Neubad*, a commodious stone building, completed in 1880, at a cost of 165,600 florins exclusive of the cost of the ground. On the ground-floor are twenty-two peat baths, and on the first floor twenty-four mineral baths, the first-class baths being of porcelain, and the second-class of wood.

Opposite the Neubad is the *Zweite Volksschule*, in the upper storey of which is the *Town Library* and *Museum*, open Wednesdays and Saturdays, 2 to 4 P.M. The Museum contains collections of natural history, minerals, and a few curiosities.

On a small eminence above the Markt Platz is the oldest building in Carlsbad, the *Stadtthurm*, or Town-tower, erected in 1608 on the site of the castle built by Charles IV. in 1358. It was greatly damaged by fire in 1757, and rebuilt a few years later. Formerly all guests arriving at Carlsbad were welcomed by a flourish of trumpets sounded from the town tower. This custom was abolished in 1852, as visitors began to complain about their rest being constantly disturbed at all hours.

In the Markt Platz is a monument to the *Holy*

Trinity, erected in 1716 by the Countess Wrtby, in commemoration of the escape of Carlsbad from the plague, which raged throughout Bohemia in 1713. In former times on Trinity Sunday the clergy of the town marched round the statue in procession after morning service.

Nearly opposite the statue is the *Post and Telegraph Office*, erected in 1875. (For post and telegraph regulations see p. 80.)

The most beautiful public building in Carlsbad is the new *Theatre* on the Neue Wiese, a handsome edifice of Renaissance architecture, with a fine façade decorated with groups of figures representing Poetry and Music, and richly ornamented with designs in terra-cotta and plaster-work. The building—which was erected in a remarkably short space of time, the first stone having been laid on the 1st of November 1885, and the first performance given on the 15th of May 1886—occupies the site of the old theatre erected in 1784. The interior is chastely decorated in white and gold in Louis XVI. style, the balcony panels being richly upholstered in red velvet. On the ceiling are four fine frescoes. The whole theatre is lighted with electric light, and the body of the house is protected from fire by an iron curtain. On the first and second floor are refreshment buffets. (For hours of performance and prices of seats see page 59.)

CHURCHES.—The principal church in Carlsbad is the Church of *St. Magdalen* or the *Dekanal Kirche*, a plain Romanesque edifice with two towers, erected in 1733-36 on the site of an older building which had fallen into great disrepair, and which was pulled down by desire of the Emperor Charles VI., who made a first donation of 1000 ducats towards the new building.

It is not known when the original church was founded, the church records having been destroyed during the great fire of 1604. The earliest mention of it, however, in existing records is in 1419.

Like the exterior, the interior is plain, and contains little of either antiquarian or artistic interest. Above the high altar is a picture of St. Magdalen, which was presented by Lord Odo Russell, the late British Ambassador at the Court of Berlin, who lived for some time at Carlsbad, and became a great favourite in the town. To the left is a painting representing the conversion of St. Magdalen, and on the right the Crucifixion with St. Magdalen at the Cross. Above the altar are four colossal figures of the Evangelists.

The services in the church are performed by the deacons of the ancient Order of the Red Cross with the Star, which was established during the Crusades to care for the sick and wounded. On their return from Palestine in 1227 they settled in Bohemia, and were presented with a hospital in Prague by King Wencelaus I., which is still under their charge. They were admitted to Holy Orders by Pope Gregory IX., and have since supplied ministers to many of the Bohemian churches. The Order still holds considerable possessions in Austria and Bohemia.

The *Andreas Kirche* in the Pragerstrasse, dating from 1500, is the oldest ecclesiastical building in Carlsbad. Over the altar is a fine painting of the martyrdom of St. Andreas, which is attributed to Leonardo da Vinci. It was the gift of Countess Pauline von Luxenstein in 1677. A copy of this picture is in the Belvedere at Vienna. In the disused graveyard attached to the church, a son of Mozart, who died at Carlsbad in 1844, is buried.

Hours of Service in the Roman Catholic Churches.— Mass daily at 7, 9, and 10 A.M. Sundays and festivals, mass, 7 and 8 A.M. High mass with sermon, 9 A.M. Mass, 11 A.M Vespers, 3 P.M.

The German Protestant Church in the Marienbadstrasse is a plain building consecrated in 1865. The church was erected by subscriptions collected among the Curguests, among whom the King of Prussia and King George of Hanover were liberal subscribers. Services on Sundays at 11 A.M. Pastor Rodewald.

The Russian Church, Marienbadstrasse, was erected in 1867. Services from May 1st to September 30th —Sundays and festivals, 11 A.M. and 6 P.M.

The English Church on the Schlossberg, a tastefully designed Gothic edifice, was consecrated by the Lord Bishop of London in 1877. Services from 1st May to 30th September—Sundays 11 A.M. and 4 P.M. The services are performed by visiting clergymen of the Church of England.

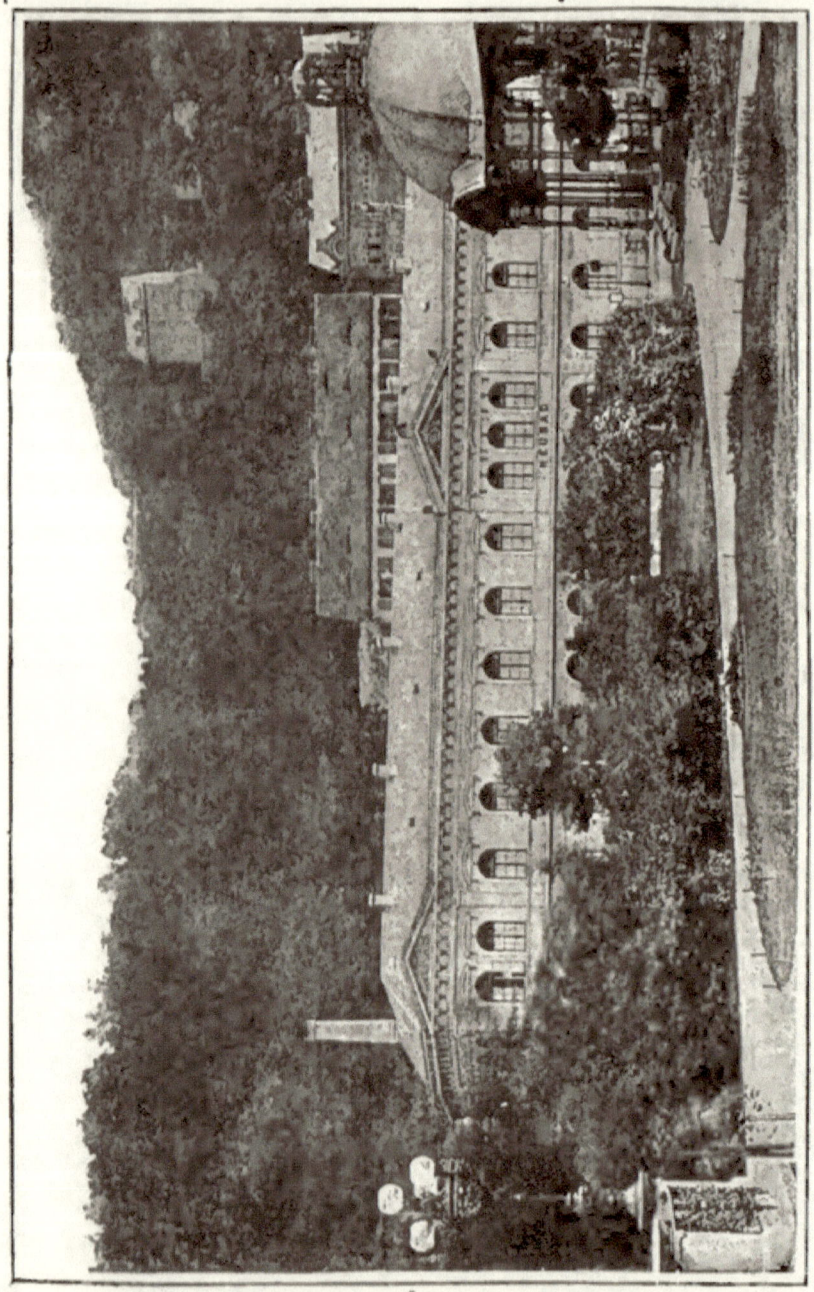

IX.

THE SPRINGS OF CARLSBAD.

TRADITION tells us that the method in which the Emperor Charles IV. took his bath was by sitting on a stone bench, carved out of the rock, over the Kaiser Karlsquelle, with his legs in the water. For the first two centuries after the discovery of the springs the waters were only used for bathing. During this period the patient was kept in the hot mineral water for eight to twelve hours at a time, the object being to cause an eruption to break out over the whole body, in order that the "evil humours," as they were called, might be brought to the surface; or, as we are told, "the waters bit the skin so that the evil matter might come out." When this took place the patient was pronounced in a fair way to recovery. It was not until 1550 that the patients began to drink the waters. This treatment was advocated by Dr. Payer in a pamphlet published in 1522, in which he writes—"Nature has created this bath for patients and not for anybody's lust or amusement." The new treatment at first seems to have been as heroic as the old, as Dr. Hoffmann, a celebrated physician of his time (1705), prescribed a dose of eighteen to twenty glasses of the water as a commencement, which was gradually increased to thirty or forty glasses. Dr. Tilling (1756), who was himself under treatment, states that he drank from fifty to sixty glasses within two hours. At that time drinking was not done, as at present, in the open air at the springs, but in a warm room, and the effect was similar to that of drinking water in a Turkish bath. When the drinking of the waters was first instituted it was alternated with the bathing—seven days being devoted to drinking, and the next seven days to the baths; but as time went on the latter period was gradually diminished and the former extended, till finally both the waters and the baths were taken together. In 1766 the first really scientific analysis of the physical and chemical properties of the mineral waters was made by Dr. David Becher, who published a pamphlet embodying his analysis and setting forth his treatment, which may be said to have been the first work which attracted general attention to the springs of Carlsbad.

The first document setting forth the virtues of the mineral waters at Carlsbad is a fine Latin Ode written by Dr. von Bohuslaw of Lobkowitz in 1510.

The theory of the rising of the springs may be generally explained as follows. The rain water and melting snow, and probably part of the river Tepel and its tributary streams, percolating through the crevices of the strata of granite rocks which underlie the district, absorb a number of mineral constituents—carbonate of soda, lime, and magnesia, sulphate of soda and potash, chloride of sodium, &c. The celebrated chemist Herr Göttl, by a series of exhaustive experiments, has proved conclusively that the granite of which the hills round Carlsbad are formed contains all the mineral constituents which have been found in the springs. These waters penetrate to a great depth, which, from the temperature of the springs, is ascertained to be not less than 8000 feet. By the action of the earth's heat at this depth on these mineral constituents, carbonic acid gas is given off, which forces the water back again to the surface, the hottest spring being that which has the shortest channel connecting it with the main reservoir. This spring is the Sprudel, but all the other springs in Carlsbad come from the same source. The taste of all the waters,—which are free from smell and not unpleasant, having been compared to the flavour of over-salted chicken broth,—is the same, except that the cooler waters contain rather more carbonic acid gas. When exposed to the air the waters become cloudy and precipitate a brown substance, which is precisely of the same nature as the Sprudelstein. The daily discharge of the springs is 2,000,000 gallons, of which two-thirds is discharged by the Sprudel.

Physical and Chemical Properties of the Springs.

Analyses of the springs have been made by Dr. Berger (1708), Dr. Borries (1733), Dr. Becher (1770), Dr. Schneider (1855), Herr Raysky (1862), Herr Göttl (1870), and by Professor Ludwig and Dr. Mauthner (1879). Their leading constituents, *sulphate of soda*, *carbonate of soda*, and *muriate of soda*, place them among the so-called alkaline and saline springs, or Glauber salt waters.

A comparative analysis of nearly all the springs has been frequently made, as above mentioned, in order to ascertain the similarity or the difference which the springs may show in their composition. It will be readily seen on examining the following table, showing the results obtained by Professor Ludwig in 1879 of the three chief springs, that their constituents are almost identical:—

Leading Constituents of the Waters.

10,000 Grammes of the Water contain	Sprudel. Temp. 162° F.	Mühlbrunn. Temp. 132° F.	Schlossbrunn. Temp. 126° F.
	Grammes.	Grammes.	Grammes.
Sulphate of soda	24.05	23.91	23.16
Carbonate of soda	12.98	12.79	12.28
Chloride of sodium	10.42	10.23	10.05
Carbonate of lime	3.21	3.27	3.34
Carbonate of magnesia	1.67	1.61	1.61
Sulphate of potash	0.86	1.19	1.93
Total of solid constituents	55.17	54.73	53.30
Carbonic acid half combined	7.76	7.68	7.49
Carbonic acid free	1.90	5.17	5.82

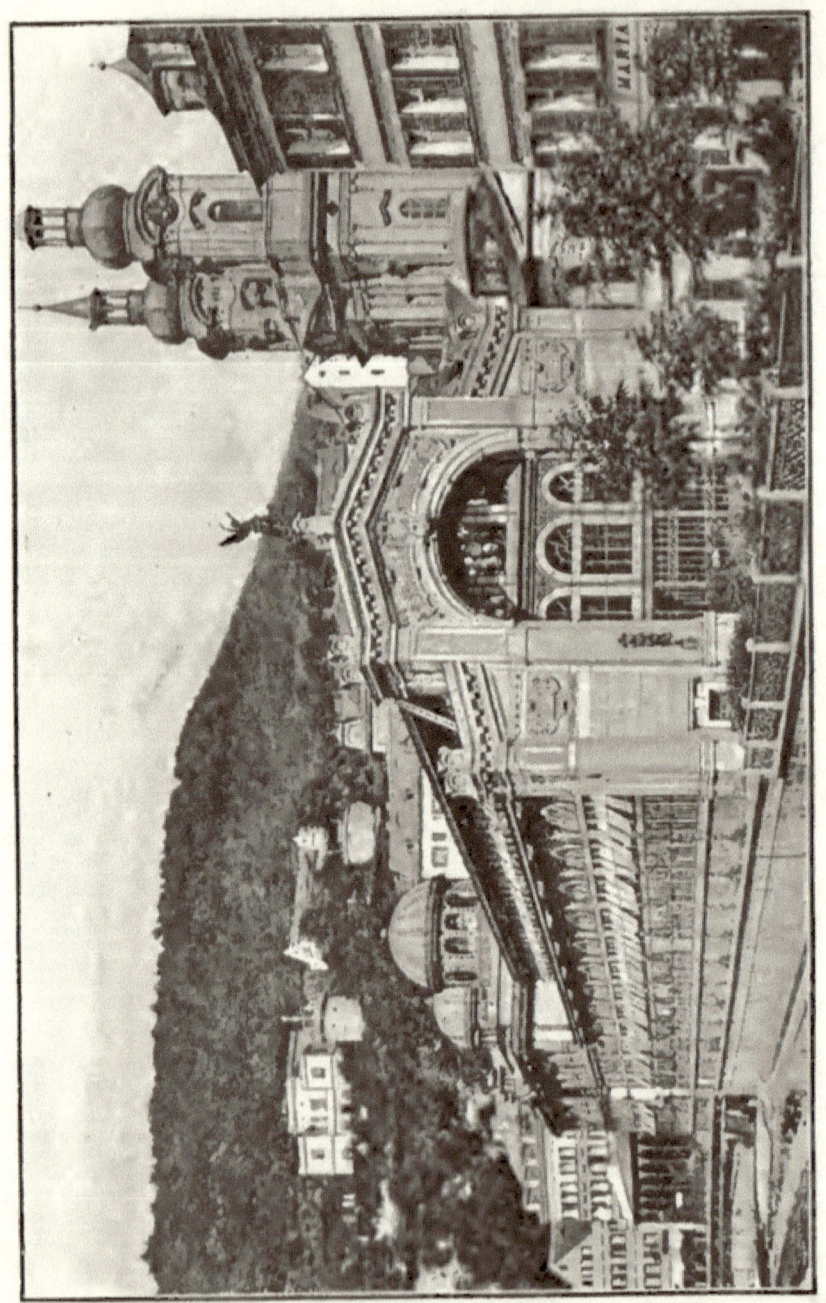

SPRUDEL COLONNADE.

Later analysis has revealed some other constituents, but only in very small quantities, namely, carbonate of iron, oxydulate of manganese, phosphate of alumina, phosphate of lime, fluoride of potassium, iodide and bromide of sodium, lithium, boracic acid, rubidium, cæsium, and arsenic.

The temperature of the springs is as follows:—

	Fahrenheit.	Réaumeur.
1. *Sprudel* } have a temperature of	166°	59.5°
2. *Hygiensquelle*		
3. *Bernhardsbrunn*	151°	53°
4. *Curhausquelle*	149°	52°
5. *Neubrunn*	145°	50°
6. *Felsenquelle*	140°	48°
7. *Theresienbrunn*	140°	48°
8. *Mühlbrunn*	133°	45°
9. *Schlossbrunn*	130°	43.5°
10. *Marktbrunn*	122°	40°
11. *Kaiserbrunn*	120°	39°
12. *Elisabethquelle*	116°	37.6°
13. *Hochbergerquelle*	106°	33°
14. *Kaiser Carlquelle*	102°	31°
15. *Russische Kronenquelle*	97°	29°
16. *Sprudelsäuerling*	84°	23°

Eleven only of these springs are now prescribed by physicians, viz., (1.) *The Sprudel*; (2.) *The Bernhardsbrunn*; (3.) *The Neubrunn*; (4.) *The Felsenquelle*; (5.) *The Theresienbrunn*; (6.) *The Mühlbrunn*; (7.) *The Schlossbrunn*; (8.) *The Marktbrunn*; (9.) *The Kaiserbrunn*; (10.) *The Elisabethquelle*; (11.) *The Kaiser Carlquelle*.

THE SPRUDEL is the most abundant and the most used

of the Carlsbad springs. It discharges about 90 gallons per minute, or 130,000 gallons per day. The waters are used both for drinking and bathing, and also for the manufacture of Sprudel salts. This spring has the property of rapidly encrusting any objects placed in it, with a thick yellowish brown coating, called sprudelstein, consisting principally of lime and silicious earth, the yellow colour being due to a small quantity of iron which it contains. The water is so impregnated with this earth that the pipes which conduct it to the surface have to be cleaned four times a year. The explanation of this phenomenon is that the mineral constituents in the water are held in solution by the carbonic acid gas. As soon as the water comes into contact with the air, it discharges its gas and precipitates the solid matter it contains. In addition to this sprudelstein, a greenish mould is formed at the edge of the springs, which, on microscopic examination, has been found to consist of animalculæ of a very low order. The waters are conducted from the main reservoir to the surface by iron pipes, which are about 20 feet in depth. Only about one-sixth of the water in the spring is discharged in the fountain, the remainder supplying the various bath-houses and the factory of the Sprudel salts, any excess of the amount required for these purposes being allowed to escape into the Tepel. The water rises in a volume about $1\frac{1}{2}$ ft. in diameter and 3 ft. in height, and every few minutes suddenly springs up to a height of 6 to 8 ft., with

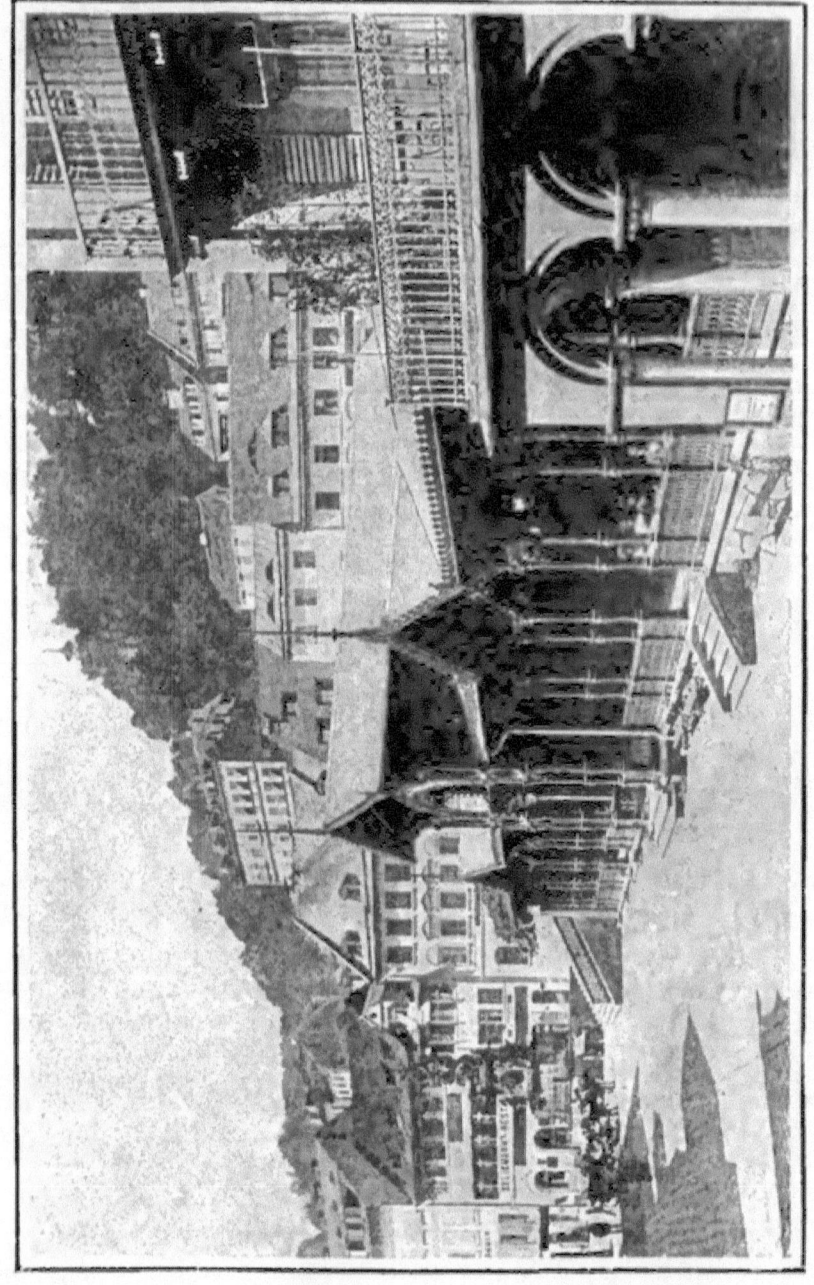

MARKTBRUNN.

a faint subterranean murmur, throwing up clouds of steam. When the volume of steam becomes excessive it is considered an almost certain sign of approaching rain. The Sprudel has a temperature of 166° Fahr., hot enough to boil eggs; indeed some of the thrifty housekeepers in the neighbourhood use the water for cooking purposes. (For analysis see page 96.) The analysis of a large body of the water made by Herr H. Göttl of Carlsbad gives traces of twenty metals and acids, of which gold is one.

There have been many violent eruptions of the Sprudel when the spring, either from an excess of steam or extra pressure of the water, has broken through the upper crust, necessitating new borings and the sealing up again of the spring. (See page .) During the great earthquake at Lisbon the spring ceased to flow for three days.

THE HYGIENSQUELLE, which springs beside the Sprudel, broke forth in 1809 during one of the eruptions of the latter spring, when it shot up in a column as high as the third storey of the neighbouring houses. Coming from the same source, its constituents are, of course, identical with those of the Sprudel. It is only used for bathing.

THE MARKTBRUNN, in the Markt Platz, enclosed in a small colonnade, was discovered in 1838, and is used for drinking. Its temperature is 122° Fahr. The following analysis was made by Dr. Ludwig of Vienna in 1879:—

In 10,000 grammes of water—

	Grammes.
Sulphate of potass	1.814
,, ,, soda	23.860
Chloride of sodium	10.304
Carbonate of lithia	0.123
,, ,, soda	12.705
,, ,, lime	3.350
,, ,, magnesia	1.634
,, ,, strontium	0.004
,, ,, protoxide of iron	0.006
,, ,, ,, ,, manganese	0.002
Borate of soda	0.040
Oxide of alumina	0.007
Phosphate of lime	0.007
Fluor of sodium	0.051
Silica	0.712
	54.619
Carbonic acid in combination	7.681
Free carbonic acid	5.557
Density	1.00357

THE KAISER KARLSQUELLE is also in the Markt Platz, and has been enclosed since 1871. It is principally used for drinking. This is the oldest spring in Carlsbad, and is supposed to have been that in which the Emperor Charles IV. bathed.

THE SCHLOSSBRUNN, discovered in 1789, is a short distance up the hill, beyond the Kaiser Karlsquelle.

This spring suddenly disappeared on the occasion of the outbreak of the Sprudel in 1809, and did not make its reappearance till 1823. The waters are principally used for drinking. (For analysis see page 96.) Opposite the Schlossbrunn is the

RUSSISCHE KRONEQUELLE, discovered in 1844, and enclosed in the Hotel Russische Krone.

The following springs are under the Mühlbrunn Colonnade:—

THE MÜHLBRUNN, known since 1571, and one of the most used of the springs. Near it is the

NEUBRUNN, which, in spite of its name, has been known for three centuries. It was first recommended in 1748 by Dr. Springsfeld, who gave it this name. It has latterly fallen into disuse, it is supposed from the absurd notion that drinking it was apt to produce vertigo. Up to 1748 the spring was only used for the treatment of sick horses. The following is the analysis by Dr. Ludwig of Vienna in 1879:—

In 10,000 grammes of water—

		Grammes.
Sulphate of potass	. . . .	1.839
,, ,, soda	. . . .	23.654
Chloride of sodium	. . . .	10.309
Carbonate of lithia	. . . .	0.113
,, ,, soda	. . . .	12.910
,, ,, lime	. . . .	3.287
,, ,, magnesia	. . . .	1.592
,, ,, strontium	. . . .	0.004

	Grammes.
Carbonate of protoxide of iron	0.026
,, ,, ,, ,, manganese	traces
Borate of soda	0.036
Oxide of alumina	0.006
Phosphate of lime	0.004
Fluor of sodium	0.046
Silica	0.709
	54,535
Carbonic acid in combination	7.627
Free carbonic acid	4.372
Density	1.00534
Temperature 145° Fahr.	

THE BERNHARDSBRUNNEN, which takes its name from statue of St. Bernhard beside it, is also but little used.

At the back of the Colonnade is the THERESIENBRUNNEN, which has been used since 1571. During the great eruption of the Sprudel in 1809 this spring ceased to flow for two days. The following is the analysis by Dr. Ludwig of Vienna in 1879:—

In 10,000 grammes of water—

	Grammes.
Sulphate of potass	1.905
,, ,, soda	23.774
Chloride of sodium	10.278
Carbonate of lithia	0.113
,, ,, soda	12.624
,, ,, lime	3.277

CARLSBAD—MÜHLBRUNN COLONNADE.

THE SPRINGS OF CARLSBAD.

	Grammes.
Carbonate of magnesia	1.577
,, ,, strontium	0.003
,, ,, protoxide of iron	0.017
,, ,, ,, ,, manganese	0.002
Borate of soda	0.036
Oxide of alumina	0.005
Phosphate of lime	0.009
Fluor of sodium	0.046
Silica	0.718
	54.384
Carbonic acid in combination	7.584
Free carbonic acid	5.100
Density	1.00537

Temperature 140° Fahr.

The ELISABETHQUELLE was discovered in 1874. Temperature, 116° Fahr. This is the coolest of the springs in general use. The following is the analysis by Dr. Ludwig of Vienna in 1879:—

In 10,000 grammes of water—

	Grammes.
Sulphate of potass	1.840
,, ,, soda	23.769
Chloride of sodium	10.314
Carbonate of lithia	0.121
,, ,, soda	12.799
,, ,, lime	3.273
,, ,, magnesia	1.642

	Grammes.
Carbonate of strontium	0.004
,, ,, protoxide of iron	0.026
,, ,, ,, ,, manganese	0.002
Borate of soda	0.030
Oxide of alumina	0.006
Phosphate of lime	0.007
Fluor of sodium	0.057
Silica	0.724
	54.614
Carbonic acid in combination	7.697
Free carbonic acid	6.085
Density	1.00539

Beyond the Mühlbrunn Colonnade is the FELSENQUELLE, which came into use in 1844, and is one of the favourite drinking springs. The following is the analysis by Dr. Ludwig of Vienna in 1879:—

In 10,000 grammes of water—

	Grammes.
Sulphate of potass	1.803
,, ,, soda	23.785
Chloride of sodium	10.314
Carbonate of lithia	0.116
,, ,, soda	12.836
,, ,, lime	3.293
,, ,, magnesia	1.615
,, ,, strontium	0.003
,, ,, protoxide of iron	0.026

THE SPRINGS OF CARLSBAD.

	Grammes.
Carbonate of protoxide of manganese	0.002
Borate of soda	0.036
Oxide of alumina	0.003
Phosphate of lime	0.007
Fluor of sodium	0.060
Silica	0.707
	54.606
Carbonic acid in combination	7.704
Free carbonic acid	4.653
Density	1.00540
Temperature 140° Fahr.	

Opposite the Curhaus is the CURHAUSQUELLE, enclosed since 1866, and principally used for bathing. The analysis made by Herr Göttl in 1872 is as follows:—

In 16 ounces = 7680 grains—

	Grains.
Sulphate of potass	1.920
,, ,, soda	18.217
Chloride of sodium	8.303
Carbonate of soda	9.002
,, ,, lime	2.459
,, ,, magnesia	1.537
,, ,, protoxide of iron	0.023
Phosphate of alumina	0.011
Silica	0.469
	41.941
Free carbonic acid	·5

THE SPRINGS OF CARLSBAD.

The KAISERBRUNNEN was discovered in 1851, in excavating the foundations of the Military Hospital, to which it is now attached. It is open to the public for drinking up to 9 o'clock in the morning, after which it is used for the baths in the hospital. The analysis made by Dr. Ludwig of Vienna in 1879 is as follows:—

In 10,000 grammes of water—

	Grammes.
Sulphate of potass	1.796
,, ,, soda	23.411
Chloride of sodium	10.103
Carbonate of lithia	0.121
,, ,, soda	12.674
,, ,, lime	3.173
,, ,, magnesia	1.602
,, ,, strontium	0.004
,, ,, oxide of iron	0.029
,, ,, ,, ,, manganese	0.002
Borate of soda	0.056
Oxide of alumina	0.005
Phosphate of lime	0.007
Fluor of sodium	0.053
Silex	0.729
	53.765
Carbonic acid in combination	7.581
Free carbonic acid	5.641
Density	1.00537

Temperature 120° Fahr.

The Eisenquelle is situated on the brow of the hill on the right bank of the Tepel, a short distance beyond the stone bridge. Though known for several centuries, it was only first used in 1852. This spring, rising from a separate source, differs entirely in its constituents from the other waters of Carlsbad. It is classed among the chalybeate springs, and is recommended in the treatment of diseases requiring iron waters. On coming to the surface the water is clear, but on being exposed to the air it takes a slight yellowish tinge. Its temperature is only 48° Fahr., which it retains even in the hottest weather. The following is the analysis by Herr Göttl in 1852:—

In 7680 grains of water—

	Grains.
Sulphate of potass	0.076
,, ,, soda	0.156
Chloride of sodium	0.152
Carbonate of soda	0.092
,, ,, lime	0.215
,, ,, magnesia	0.053
Phosphate of iron	0.008
Oxide of iron	0.345
Silica	0.013
Organic matter	0.268
	1.378
Carbonic acid	1.300 to 1.700.

The waters are used both for drinking and bathing.

The Sauerbrunn rises behind the Dorotheenau. It contains but few mineral ingredients, but is largely impregnated with carbonic acid gas, and is an agreeable and refreshing drinking water. It is also used for bathing. Its temperature varies between 53° and 60° Fahr.

X.

WALKS.

The letters and numbers in brackets refer to the numbers on the plan in the pocket at the end of the volume. These numbers are also plainly marked, for the guidance of visitors, on trees or rocks at the sides of the paths.

To the Alte Wiese, Kiesweg, Posthof, and Kaiser Park.

THE most frequented and one of the most beautiful promenades at Carlsbad is the *Alte Wiese*, "Old Meadow," which commences from the market-place and follows the left bank of the Tepel up the valley. The Alte Wiese, which is beautifully shaded with chestnut trees, presents an animated scene in the season, when it is thronged by all classes of visitors, who assemble here twice a day to promenade and to sit under the trees drinking their coffee and listening to the strains of the band at the Café Pupp. On the left-hand side, as far as the Café Pupp, and on the river-side as far as the second bridge, the street is lined with good shops, giving it the appearance of a bazaar. At the farther end, in the *Pupp'sche Allée*, is the handsome *Hotel* and *Café Pupp*, at which the band plays thrice weekly. The open space in front of the Café is planted with trees, under which are placed tables and chairs for the accommodation of visitors. In the Café is a large and handsome salon, in which the band plays when the weather is unfavourable.

Beyond the Pupp'sche Allée we come to the *Kiesweg* (C 1), a beautifully shaded avenue which leads along the river up the valley as far as the *Kaiser-Brücke* (C 11). We first pass the fine marble monument of *Goethe*, unveiled in 1883. The monument, the first erected to Goethe in Austria, cost 12,000 marks. To the right, above a little grotto, is the *Rasumowska Platz*, an open space with seats, named in honour of the Russian Countess Rasumowska. The rocks on the side of the road here are covered with inscriptions recording the gratitude of many visitors, high and low, for the benefits they have received from the Carlsbad waters. We next pass on the right hand the *Rohan Platz* (C 6), a little shady nook with an iron table and seats, which were placed here by the family of the present Prince de Rohan, who has made forty-two visits to Carlsbad. On the trunk of a beech-tree we read an inscription to the memory of his father, the late Prince Louis de Rohan (d. 1837). Adjoining the Rohan Platz is the *Kaizerin Sitz*, "Empress's Seat," erected in memory of its having been the favourite resting-place of the Austrian

Empress, Maria Ludovika (the third wife of Francis I.), who visited Carlsbad in 1810. Goethe has celebrated the erection of this Sitz in some charming verses. On the heights above the Sitz is the *Summer Theatre* (page 61).

We now reach the *Sans Souci* (C 8), an elegant café, with a concert salon and tables under the trees. On the opposite side of the river is the little *Dorotheen's Temple* (Cd 12), erected in honour of the Herzogin Dorothee in 1791. A few steps farther bring us to a small rock called the *Paulinen Sitz*, dedicated to Pauline, Duchess of Hohenzollern. From this rock there is a most picturesque view of the romantic valley of the Tepel.

The Kiesweg ends at the *Karlsbrücke* (C 11), an iron bridge of one arch crossing the Tepel, erected in 1880 at a cost of 29,000 fl. The first bridge here was simply a wooden foot-bridge, waggons and carriages having to cross the river over a ford. This bridge was replaced in 1798 by a carriage-bridge, which was carried away by a flood in 1801. A third bridge was then erected and opened by Maria Theresa, who named it the Karlsbrücke in honour of her brother, the Grand Duke Charles, the victor of Aspern. After this the bridge was several times destroyed by floods, lastly in 1821, when the heavy wooden beams, being carried down the river, did immense damage, breaking into the houses and carrying away a number of the bridges lower down. In 1822 the Town

Council resolved to build an iron bridge, and began to collect subscriptions for this purpose; but it was not until 1880 that the bridge was finally completed.

Beyond the Karlsbrücke the valley widens considerably and takes a sharp bend to the south, forming a picturesque amphitheatre, surrounded by beautifully wooded hills, rising abruptly from the level meadows. Here we come to the *Vier Uhr Promenade* (Ca 11), " Four o'clock Promenade "—so called from its being in the shade after 4 P.M.—a beautifully shaded avenue which leads up to the right to the *Fürstenstein-Sitz*, " Princesses Seat " (Ca 12), a small platform of rock named in honour of Queen Pauline of Würtemburg, the Archduchess Maria of Austria, and the Duchess Amelia of Sachsen-Altenburg, three royal sisters who often visited Carlsbad. The names of the princesses are engraved in gilt letters on a black marble tablet. Farther on is the *Schwarzenberg Monument* (Ca 14), a pyramid erected in honour of Field-Marshal Prince von Schwarzenberg, the conqueror of Leipzic, by some officers of the Austrian army.

On the right of the Karlsbrücke are a number of shooting-galleries, which are largely patronised by visitors. In the meadow is a granite *obelisk*, erected in 1883, as a thank-offering, by several Hungarian patients who were cured at Carlsbad. To the left, on the brow of the hill, are the *Sauerbrunn* baths and drinking-hall (see p. 108). Above the Sauerbrunn is the *Café Schweizerhof*, and farther along the brow of the hill the *Café Schönbrunn*, two favourite resorts in summer. From both the Kiesweg and the Vier Uhr Promenade well-laid-out paths lead up the hills through the woods, the directions being indicated everywhere by finger-posts.

Following the main road, which is lined with poplar trees, and which follows the course of the Tepel, affording beautiful glimpses of river and woodland scenery, we reach the *Café Posthof*, with a prettily laid out garden, where Labitzky's band plays on Mondays, Wednesdays, and Fridays from 4 to 6 P.M., the concerts on Friday being symphony concerts (entrance 50 kr.) The large concert salon, called the "Prussian Hall," was opened in 1817 with a ball, given in honour of Marshal Blücher by the Cur-guests. From the Posthof an avenue of fruit-trees leads up the hill on the right to the *Schwarzenberg Sitz* (see above).

Beyond the Café Posthof the course of the valley turns westward, and, continuing our walk, we next pass on the right the *Antons Ruhe* (C 22), named in honour of King Anthony of Saxony. Here a path to the left, leading to Pirkenhammer, crosses the river over a foot-bridge. About ten minutes farther on we come to the *Freundschaft's-Salle* (C 31) or "Friendship's Salon," a favourite resort, with a good restaurant and café, erected in 1819–23. The Salle was opened with a ball given in honour of the Duchess of Cumberland. The café is surrounded by a pretty and well-shaded garden, and military concerts are given twice weekly from 4 to 6 P.M. Opposite is the *Sitz der Freunde*, "the Friends' Seat," erected in 1781, and named in honour of the Russian Admiral Orloff and Count Brühl, who were boon companions, and who often visited Carlsbad together. Five years later the Countess Brühl erected a small granite tablet with the inscription, 'À Hygeia le XXI. Août MDCCLXXXVI. erigé par Tina Brühl." Near it is another stone with the inscription, "Elle écarte les maux, les langueurs, les faiblesses, sans elle beauté n'est plus"—She drives away the evils of languor and weakness—without her beauty cannot exist.

Beyond this point the road, still following the river, again bends northwards, leading in about a quarter of an hour to the *Kaiser Park* (C 41), a Swiss chalet, with a café and restaurant nestling in a most picturesque and shady nook. The walk can be extended by following the road for half an hour to the village of Pirkenhammer (see p. 126).

To the Ecce Homo Kapelle, Franz Josef's Höhe, and Findlater's Temple.

Starting from the Pupp'sche Allée we turn to the right up the hill and reach the *Mariannen's Ruhe* (A 10), a rocky prominence surmounted by a cross, from which there is a pretty view of the Alte Wiese and the town. On the side of the rock is the inscription, "Plus être que paraître"—"Be more than you appear to be." This spot is named in honour of the Princess Marian of Saxony. From the Mariannen's Ruhe we take the *Buturlin Weg* (following the marks Ab), a road constructed by the Russian Count Buturlin, which ascends through the wood in about twenty minutes to the *Hammer* or *Ecce Homo Kapelle.* Here two paths, indicated by finger-posts, branch off, leading to the *Franz Josef's Höhe*, which is crowned with glorietta, commanding one of the most beautiful views round Carlsbad. Beyond the Franz Josef's Höhe we follow the path, A 29 to 12, where we again reach the Pupp'sche-Allée.

Another path (B) from the Ecce Homo Chapel descends to the *Findlater's Temple,* a classical semi-circular building surrounded by a cupola, erected by Lord Findlater, a Scotch nobleman, in gratitude for the benefits he received from the Carlsbad waters.

Beyond the Findlater's Temple a path descends on the right (Ca 28–39) to the *Freundschaft's Salle* (p. 113), the main path (Ca 28–15) leading to the Schwartzenberg Obelisk and the Vier Uhr Promenade (p. 112).

To the Findlater's Pyramid and Freundschaft's-Höhe.

Starting from the Mariennen's Ruhe (A 10), near the Pupp'sche Allée (see page 109), we take the first path to the right (Ab 11), which leads in windings through the wood, passing the *Helenen's Sitz*, the favourite resting-place of the Grand Duchess Helena of Russia, to the *Findlater's Pyramid*, a granite obelisk, twenty-eight feet in height, erected in 1804 in honour of Lord Findlater, "the friend and beautifier of nature, as a token of the gratitude of the citizens of Carlsbad." The pyramid commands a fine view of the valley below.

About a quarter of an hour farther up the hill (by path D) we come to the *Freundschaft's-Höhe* (D 5), also commanding a beautiful view. From here a small footpath ascends to the *Vogelhütte*, the highest point on the left bank of the river with the exception of the Aberg. From the Freundschaft's-Höhe we descend to the *Friedrich Wilhelm Platz*, named in honour of Frederick William III., from which there is one of the finest views of the town. A little lower down (path W) is an open space in the wood, which is often illuminated. From here a path winds down to the *Marien Kapelle*, behind the Hotel Pupp.

To the Hirschensprung.

The easiest way of making the ascent of the Hirschensprung is by starting from the Markt Platz or Curhaus and ascending to the English chapel, where we take the road to the left (B 5). After passing the mark B 8, we find a path to the left, called the *Jubiläumsweg*, which leads to the *Himmel auf Erden*, a little retired spot which scarcely merits its high-sounding name. Beyond this we take a path to the right, shortly after passing Jb 2, which joins the path, described below, leading directly up to the Hirschensprung. The rocks here are covered with inscriptions commemorating cures by the Carlsbad waters.

A shorter but somewhat steeper path can be taken from the Markt Platz by passing the Schlossbrunnen and turning to the left along the Hirschensprunggasse, from which a path (at A 5) turns to the right, leading in windings up the face of the hill. At Aa 8 the path divides, and we take that leading to the right, which shortly after joins the path from the Jubiläumsweg (see above). A short distance farther on the path divides, leading on the right directly to the restaurant, and to the left to *Meyer's Gloriette*, a little temple built by a merchant of Vienna who was a native of Carlsbad. Near this point is an isolated rock, on the summit of which is a bronze figure of a chamois. Beyond the Gloriette we pass a black marble tablet erected in honour of the Grand Duke of Saxe Weimar, and reach the *Petershöhe*, named in honour of Peter the Great, who ascended the Hirschensprung mounted on a bare-backed horse, and inscribed on the cross the letters, M. S. P. I., " Manu sua Petrus I." This cross has unfortunately been destroyed, the present cross, which is on the summit of the rock, being modern. On the rock before the cross is a colossal bust of Peter the Great. On the face of the rock below is a black marble slab on which are inscribed the names of Russian nobles who have visited Carlsbad, the list being headed by the name of Peter the Great. A few steps above the Petershöhe is the *Theresienhöhe*, a small open space with a stone pryamid erected in honour of Theresa of Angoulême. A stone stairway now leads us to the summit of the Hirschensprung, which commands a magnificent panoramic view of the valleys of the Tepel and Eger and the Erzgebirge. A short distance below the summit, on a terrace, is a café restaurant.

The Hirschensprung, or Deer's Leap, is the traditional spot from which the deer sprang while pursued by Charles IV. (see page 28).

To the Belvidere and Aberg.

Starting up the hill from the Marien Kapelle behind the Café Pupp, and passing the *Friedrich Wilhelm Platz* (see page 116), we take the path to the right at B 20, and then to the left at B 19, along the brow of the hill, keeping the Freundschaft's Höhe (see page 116) on our right, and after a pleasant walk of about twenty minutes through the woods we arrive at the *Katharinen Platz* (E 9), a sheltered nook among the trees, named in Leopold Stöhr's "Reminiscences of Carlsbad," after his friend Katharine Deimel. A short distance beyond, a path to the left (Ea 13) leads up to the *Belvidere*, which commands a fine view of the valley, with the ruins of Engelhaus in the distance. Near the Belvidere the path (G) descends to the Kaiser Park (see page 114). If, instead of turning off to the Belvidere at E 13, we keep straight on, we come to the *Bild*, so called from a picture of the Madonna fastened to a pine-tree. In about twenty minutes more, keeping along the path E, we reach the summit of the *Aberg*, 2000 feet above the sea, or 806 feet above the Sprudel, the highest point near Carlsbad. Near the summit is a café and a tower, from which we have a magnificent view. Beyond the summit the path turns northwards, and descends to Ziegelhütte, where refreshments can be had. We can return to Carlsbad by St. Leonard's Chapel and the Echo (see route below).

Another way to reach the Aberg is by taking the road from the Schlossberg, passing the English Church, and following the road B till we come to B 13, when we take the road Be, leading to *Kaiser Karl IV.'s Jägerhaus*. Passing the bowling-green, we come to an open space, and crossing a small brook, find a path on the left (at Be 24), which leads up to the *Russell Sitz*, a seat on a rock named in honour of Lord Odo Russell, the late British Ambassador to the Court of Berlin. The rock commands a fine view of the *Erzgebirge*, through an opening in the woods.

Beyond this we reach the *Echo*, a spot where an echo answers five or six times. From the Echo we take the path Beb, and next pass, situated on a small hill, the *Chapel of St. Leonard*, formerly the parish church of the ancient village of *Thiergarten*, of which only a few traces now remain of old walls built of Sprudelstein. The inhabitants of this village migrated to Carlsbad after King John had issued his charter (see page 28). The chapel has been restored by the late Lord Odo Russell, British Ambassador to the Court of Berlin. About ten minutes farther on we arrive at *Ziegelhütte*, from whence we take a path to the left, leading up to the summit of the hill (see route above).

To the Weisses Kreuz and Schützen Park.

Proceeding to the English Church, we take the road to the right (Bb), which we follow as far as the *Restaurant Klein Versailles* (Bb 12). Here we cross the meadows by a path which leads along the edge of the forest. A few paces beyond Bb 22 we turn to the right, and in about five minutes arrive at a group of rocks, surmounted by a white cross, called the *Weisses Kreuz*. Farther on, the path reaches the Marie Sophienweg, a carriage road, along which we turn first to the right (32) and then to the left (31), and winding round the slope of the mountain, have beautiful views of the valley of the Eger. We now descend into the valley, and take the road leading to the railway station, and passing the restaurant of the *Schützen Park*, return to Carlsbad.

To the Panorama, Waldschloss, Drei Kreuzberg, and Ewiges Leben.

Starting from the church opposite the Sprudel Colonnade, and proceeding up the Schulgasse to the left, we arrive first at the *Stephan's Platz*, and then reach the *Stadtgarten*, an open space in which is a column surmounted by a statue of Charles IV., erected in 1858 to commemorate the 500th anniversary of the foundation of Carlsbad. From here we have a fine view of the town. A short distance farther on, on the left, is the *Panorama*, a favourite point of view, with a café restaurant, in which is a collection of stuffed animals killed in the neighbourhood.

The return to the town can be made by following the road to the left, or the walk may be extended by taking the first road to the right from the Prager Strasse, which leads by a winding path to the villa of *Waldschloss*. The next turning to the right (K) from the Prager Strasse, a short distance before we come to the Andreas-Kirche, leads up the hill winding round behind the slope to the *Restaurant* of the Drei-Kreuzberg, with a small garden. Near the Restaurant is a *camera obscura*. Five minutes farther on we reach the summit of the *Drei-Kreuzberg* itself, and in ten minutes more the summit of the *Otto's-Höhe*, named in honour of the late King of Greece, to whom a statue has been erected.

To return from the Otto's-Höhe we can descend a

steep path which leads directly down to the Panorama. From the Otto's-Höhe a footpath leads to the summit of the Ewiges Leben (2003 feet), the highest point near Carlsbad. On the summit a gloriette has been erected, which commands the most extensive view round Carlsbad.

To the Wiener Sitz, Sauerbrunn, and Schweizerhof.

We proceed along the right bank of the Tepel by the Marienbad Strasse, passing on our right, as we approach the Karlsbrücke, on the face of a steep rock, the iron head of a lion, with a serpent in its mouth, designed and erected by the sculptor Kiess. On the face of the rock are numerous inscriptions recording cures. A little farther on is the Dorotheen's Temple erected in 1791 in honour of Dorothée, Duchess of Curland. Before arriving at the bridge we take a path (Cd) up the hill to the left, and join another path leading along the brow of the hill. Taking this path to the left (Ce) we come to the *Wiener Sitz*, an eminence commanding a fine panoramic view of the town and valley. On this point there is an elegant temple, erected in 1840 by a subscription made among the Cur-guests. Several paths lead from the west side of the Wiener Sitz directly into the town.

The path to the right, opposite the Dorotheen's

Temple, leads to the *Sauerbrunn* drinking-hall and baths, and to the *Schweizerhof*, a prettily situated restaurant, with a garden, commanding a fine view up the valley of the Tepel. From the Saurbrunn we can descend into the valley again by taking the path to the right, and crossing the river by the foot-bridge a short distance above the Karlsbrücke.

To the Schönbrunn.

We follow the Kiesweg to the Karlsbrücke, and keeping along on the road leading to the Posthof for a short distance, we take a road to the left planted with trees, and crossing the Tepel by a foot-bridge, ascend the hill opposite, to the *Restaurant Schönbrunn*. From here paths lead in all directions through the woods which overhang the right bank of the Tepel. From the Café the *Schwindelweg* follows the brow of the hill, passing the *Augusten's Platz*, on which is a pyramid, erected in 1823 in honour of the Duchess of Cumberland, finally arriving at the Kaiser Park (see p. 114). Some short distance (Cb 33) before arriving at the Kaiser Park a path descends to the right, crossing the river over a foot-bridge, reaching the Freundschaftsaal (see p. 115).

To the Veitsberg.

We follow a path turning off from the Schwindelweg (see above), nearly opposite the Posthof (see p. 113), which

ascends the hill through beautifully wooded scenery to
the summit of the *Veitsberg*. Descending on the other
side, we leave on the right the village of Espenthor,
and turning to the left again ascend, arrive at a
most picturesque little glade, surrounded by beeches,
from which we can return again to the Schwindelweg.
This walk is one of the most beautiful in the neighbourhood of Carlsbad, with its lovely and ever-chang-
ing views of the Tepel valley, and the open country on
the other side towards Engelhaus.

To the Rothe-Säuerling.

Starting from the Andreasgasse, near the Andreas-
Kirche, we take the road leading up the Galgenberg,
passing a small monument erected to commemorate
the exodus of the Protestant citizens of Carlsbad, who
left the city in 1624, in consequence of the re-establishment of the Catholic religion by Ferdinand II.
Before reaching the Cemetery we find (at O 8) a path,
rather ill-defined, leading down to the main road to
Giesshübl. From here we take another path to the
left, which brings us to the Rothe-Säuerling, a small
mineral spring. Near the bank of the Eger, a short
distance down the river, is *Eulenfels* or *Hexenfels*,
"Rock of the Owls or Witches," at which, according to
a local tradition, the witches meet on Walpurgis night,
and after having gone through their incantations ascend
the Bloxberg on their brooms. Returning, we take

the main Giesshübl road, which brings us back to Carlsbad.

To Dallwitz.

We take the Saurbrunn Strasse, the main road to Giesshübl, and come to the village of Drahowitz, where we cross the Eger in a small ferry-boat. Turning to the right, we proceed along the bank of the river for about half an hour, when we come to a small brook, which we follow for about ten minutes, till we reach *Dalwitz*, celebrated for its magnificent oak-trees, some of which are so large that it requires five or six men with outstretched arms to encircle them. At the village there is a porcelain manufactory, specimens of which are exhibited in the small castle. Refreshments can be had at the Restaurant *Zu Drei Eichen*, "Three Oaks." The return journey can be made by taking the road up the hill, crossing the railway, and joining the main road leading to the railway station at Carlsbad.

XI.

DRIVES ROUND CARLSBAD.

Hammer, Aich, and Hans Heiling-Fels.

(For omnibus to Hammer and Aich, see page 78.)

THE Hans Heiling-Fels can be reached either by the valley of the Eger or the valley of the Tepel, both roads joining at the village of Aich. The pleasantest way is to go by the valley of the Tepel and return by the Eger.

Leaving Carlsbad, we drive along the Marienbad Strasse, crossing the Tepel at the Karlsbrücke, and passing the Kaiser Park (see p. 114) reach the village of Pirkenhammer, celebrated for its wood-carving industry; it has also a large porcelain manufactory, over which visitors are shown. Behind the factory rises the *Mecseryhöhe*, from which there is a fine view of the Tepel valley. There are two good restaurants at Pirkenhammer, Leibold's and Habsburg.

A short distance beyond Pirkenhammer we leave the Tepel, and cross over into the valley of the Eger, which we reach at the village of *Aich*. At Aich there is a

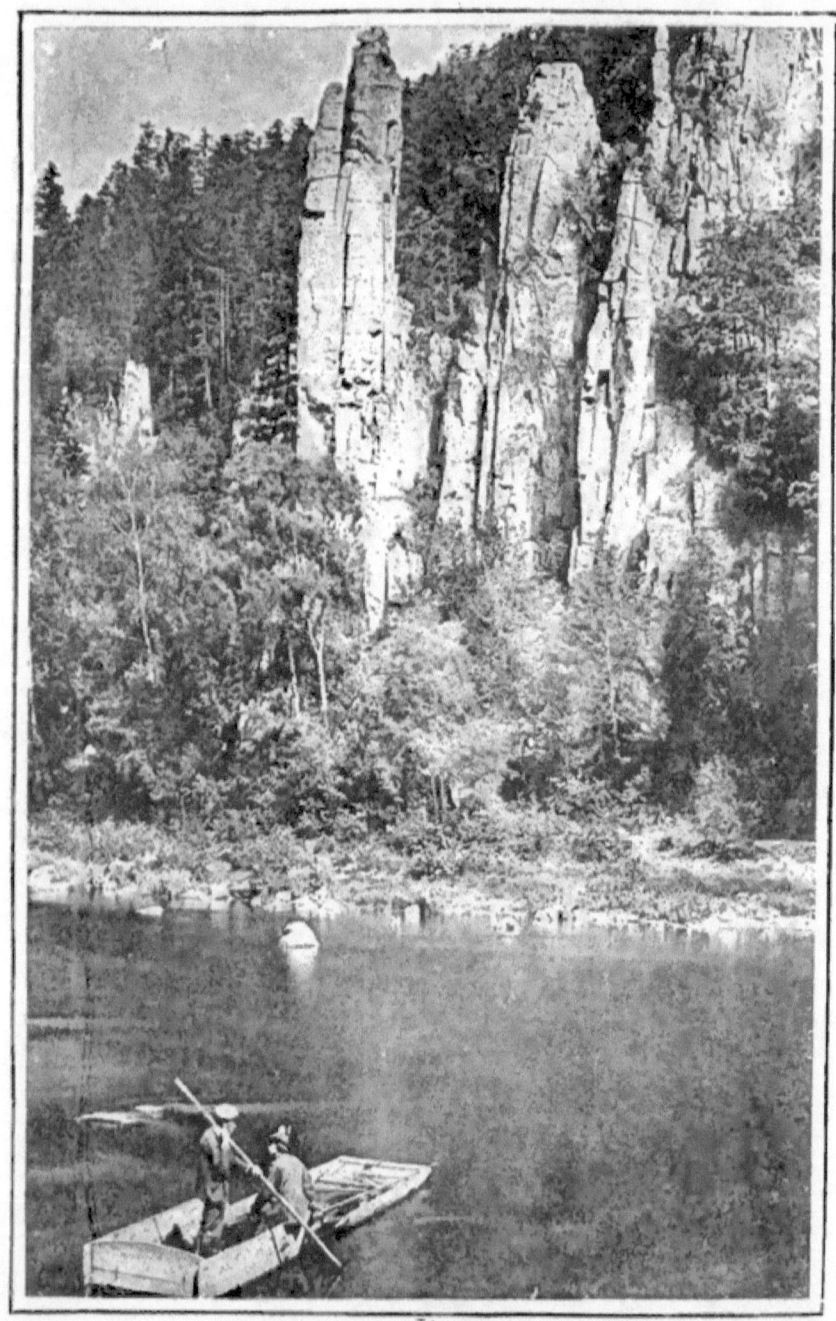

HANS HEILING-FELS.

Reproduced by permission of Amand Helm, Vienna.

little château with a café restaurant, and a porcelain manufactory with a *specialité* of photographs on china.

From Aich it is about half an hour's walk to *Hans Heiling-Fels*, a picturesque group of rocks overhanging the Eger. A romantic legend is connected with these rocks, which forms the subject of the opera of Marschener and a novel by Kröner.

Once upon a time there lived in a village in the valley of the Eger a wealthy farmer named Veit, whose only daughter, Elsbeth, was famed far and wide for her beauty and accomplishments. Near the farm, in a small hut, there lived an honest and industrious peasant, whose son Arnold was Elsbeth's favourite playfellow. As the boy grew up he developed a restless disposition and a love of adventure, and finally left home to seek his fortune in foreign lands. After an absence of several years Arnold returned to his native village only just in time to close his aged parents' eyes in death. A few days afterwards he and Elsbeth met again, and bringing back the tender recollections of the happy childhood they had spent together, they renewed their former friendship, which soon ripened into love. After plighting their troth Arnold lost no time in seeking the father of Elsbeth and requesting her hand in marriage. Veit at first received him in a friendly manner, and listened with interest to the story of his adventures in foreign lands; but as soon as Arnold touched on the subject nearest his heart the old man gave him a short and surly answer. At last, however, he promised that if

Arnold succeeded in making his way in the world during the next three years he would then give his consent to the union of the lovers. After a tender parting, in which vows of eternal constancy were exchanged, Arnold, with a heavy heart, set out once more to seek his fortune, promising that, rich or poor, he would return when the three years were past.

Now, many years before this, one of the villagers, named Hans Heiling, had mysteriously disappeared, and nothing having been heard from him, he had long since been forgotten. About a year after the departure of Arnold, Hans suddenly returned, apparently a rich and prosperous man. He had, however, became proud and morose, and many strange stories began to be circulated among the villagers, who all began to look upon him with suspicion, with the exception of Veit, with whom, by flattery and judicious presents, he had succeeded in ingratiating himself. This influence he soon began to use to further his suit with Elsbeth, of whom he had become deeply enamoured. Elsbeth, however, remained true to her lover, and rejected his advances with scorn. Finding it impossible to win her hand by fair means, Hans Heiling brought the arts of magic to his aid; but Elsbeth, who had received a friendly warning, constantly wore a small cross which her lover had given her round her neck as a talisman, and which was effectual in keeping her evil lover and his unwelcome attentions at a distance.

One day, however, the charm was stolen from Elsbeth

through the cunning of Hans, who became daily more importunate. By this time the three years of probation had nearly elapsed, and, nothing having been heard of Arnold, doubts of his fidelity began to creep into Elspeth's bosom. Worn out by the importunities of Heiling and the menaces of her father, the unhappy girl at last reluctantly gave her consent to the hated union, and the date of the marriage was fixed.

Three days now only remained of the three years, and as they slowly passed Elspeth began to waver and to bitterly repent the promise she had given. She still clung desperately to the fond hope that her young lover might even yet return in time to save her.

The morning of the last day arrived. The wedding with Heiling was to take place on the following day, and Elspeth had already given herself up as lost, when there suddenly came galloping into the village a troup of horsemen with Arnold at their head. Riding straight to the house of Elspeth's father, and hastily informing him that during his absence he had succeeded in obtaining rank and fortune, he demanded of him the fulfilment of his promise. At the same time some of Arnold's followers recognised in Hans Heiling a well-known sorcerer. Veit, on hearing this, and on seeing the good fortune of Arnold, now readily gave his consent to the union of the true lovers, who were shortly afterwards united.

After the wedding the happy couple, accompanied by their friends, adjourned to a meadow on the banks of the

Eger, where Veit had a tent erected and a supper prepared. The evening passed quickly in merriment till it was close upon midnight; but just as the last stroke of the church clock struck twelve a terrible storm of wind and rain suddenly burst on the affrighted company, and amid the darkness appeared the form of Hans Heiling, surrounded by a legion of devils and imps, his face frightfully distorted and flaming with passion. He suddenly plunged into the foaming depths of the river and disappeared; but the wedding company remained rooted to the spot, having been all changed by the power of the devil into stone; and still from the river-bank they are said to look down with melancholy countenances on the passers-by.

Returning from Aich we follow the right bank of the river Eger, passing the villages of Meiershofen and Donitz to Carlsbad.

To Engelhaus.

The drive to Engelhaus takes about two hours there and back. From Carlsbad we follow the Prager Strasse, the old coach-road to Prague, having fine views of Carlsbad and the Tepel valley. The Prager Strasse was constructed by the Emperor Francis I. in 1804, and on the portion between Carlsbad and Engelhaus shows great engineering skill. About half-way we pass on the right at the village of Berghäuser an ancient inn, the *Bergwirthshaus*, erected about the thirteenth century. Some of the walls are from 10 to 12 feet thick.

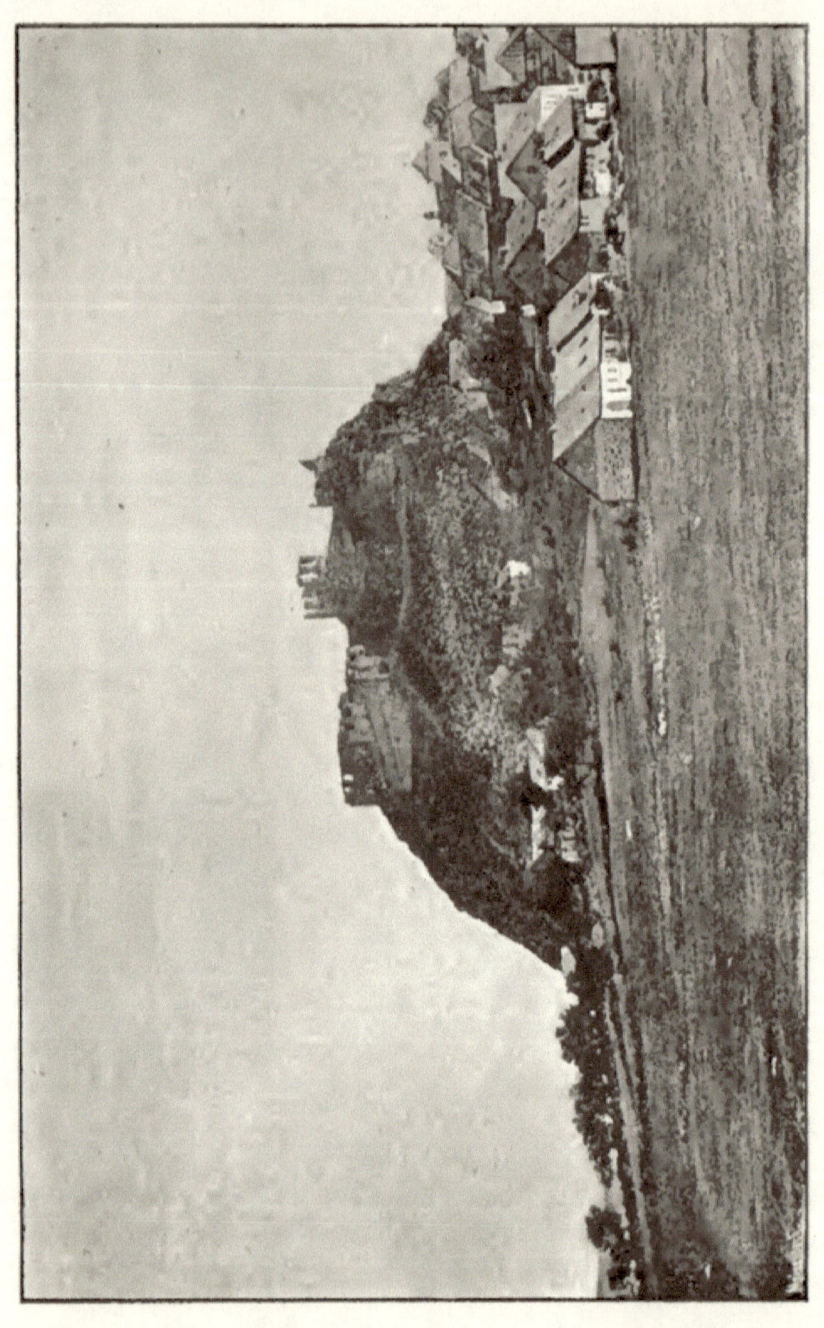

ENGELHAUS.

At *Engelhaus* there is a small inn where refreshments can be had.

The ruins of the *Castle of Engelhaus*, of which now but a few crumbling fragments remain, occupy the summit of an isolated and precipitous rock 468 feet in height, which is ascended by a dilapidated stone staircase from behind the church. The date of the building of the castle is lost in obscurity, but mention of it is made in records of the twelfth and thirteenth centuries.

Many interesting legends are told about this castle, among which the most prominent are the legend of King Arthur and the legend of Aloisia.

King Arthur one day while hunting in England was attracted by the screams of an infant. On approaching the spot he found a handsome baby boy in the claws of a bear, which had already devoured the infant's mother. The king killed the savage beast, took the child home with him, and adopted him as his son, having him baptized Richard. The boy grew up brave and handsome, and in time fell secretly in love with the king's daughter, Albina, who returned his affection. Fearing the king would forbid their union they arranged to elope, and one dark night, accompanied by a few devoted followers, fled from the royal castle. On their arrival at the sea-shore they found a ship awaiting them, in which they crossed to the coast of France, and finally, after many wanderings, reached the mountains of Bohemia in the vicinity of Engelhaus. Here, on the rock on which the ruins now stand, Richard erected a strong fortress, in which he and his wife lived in seclusion for many years.

Their marriage was blessed with many children; but their happiness was not complete, as Albina often reproached herself for her undutiful conduct towards her father. Richard also, in time, began to tire of his wife, whose beauty had begun to fade, and of the monotonous life they led. He also regretted having thrown away his chances of advancement at the English court, and as time wore on mutual reproaches followed.

Meanwhile King Arthur, who had mourned the loss of his daughter for many years, abdicated in favour of his nephew, and determined to spend the rest of his life in searching for her. He first sought the advice of an Arabian astrologer, who, by his magic arts, ascertained the hiding-place of the errant couple. Disguised in the garb of a pilgrim, and attended only by a few faithful knights, the king travelled through Germany and Bohemia until he reached a small village in the neighbourhood of Engelhaus, where he left his attendants and proceeded to the castle, to which, in his assumed character of a pilgrim, he soon obtained admission. On hearing him speak English, however, Richard began to suspect he might be a spy sent by the king, and refused him permission to see his wife, threatening at the same time, if he discovered his suspicions were true, to put him in a cauldron of boiling oil. The old king on hearing this left the castle and sought the assistance of a neighbouring knight, to whom he told his sad story. The knight in return informed him how Richard had begun to neglect his wife, and how unhappy she had become, and at the same time proffered his services to try to capture the castle and release Albina.

News of the intended attack was brought to Richard, who, in revenge, resolved to poison his wife and flee from the country. To carry out his villainous scheme he went to Albina, and pretending to have repented of his former ill-usage, proposed that they should pledge their reconciliation in a goblet of wine, and should then go together and seek the pardon of King Arthur. Two goblets of wine, one of which had been poisoned, were brought in. Handing the deadly draught to his wife, and taking the other himself, they were just about to drink the pledge when a flourish of trumpets outside proclaimed the approach of the attacking army. Albina and Richard, eager to see the old king and his followers, though from very different motives, put down their glasses untasted; but Richard, who now recognised the king, anxious to complete his treacherous design before the arrival of the besiegers, again took up the goblets, and handing one to his wife they both drank them off, and then Richard instantly made his escape. Albina rushed to meet her father, and throwing herself at his feet implored his pardon, which was only too gladly granted. He had hardly raised her from the ground when a knight rushed in, bringing the news that Richard had been found in the castle-yard expiring in mortal agony. In his haste he had unwittingly changed the glasses and drunk the fatal draught himself. After the burial of Richard, Albina returned to England, and the castle, which was afterwards haunted by the ghost of the would-be murderer, remained uninhabited for many centuries.

Another romantic legend is that of Aloisia.

Othon Sigismond, Count of Wratibor von Starkowitz-Schwarzstein, a Bohemian nobleman, who fought on the side of the French at the battle of Crecy in A.D. 1346, was dangerously wounded and taken prisoner by the English, but was afterwards released on paying a heavy ransom. During his captivity in England he wooed and married Aloisia, the beautiful Duchess of Westmoreland, grand-daughter of Edward I. After his ransom he brought her to his castle of Schwarzstein as Engelhaus was then called. For four years she lived a life of unalloyed happiness with her beloved husband, but soon after the birth of their son and heir, Sigismond was called on to join the standard of his liege lord the Emperor Charles IV. in an expedition to quell a rebellion which had broken out among the cities of Northern Italy.

Before he left he committed the care of his wife and son, and the management of his estates to his friend Count Wlanitz, who had been his fellow-prisoner in England. During their joint captivity there, Wlanitz had also been in love with Aloisia, and, though unknown to Sigismond, had tried to gain her hand. As long as Sigismond had remained to protect his wife Wlanitz had kept his passion under due control, but no sooner did he find her alone and in his power than he renewed his protestations of love. The Countess, faithful to her husband, rejected his advances with scorn, till, maddened by his passion, Wlanitz determined on a bitter revenge. Intercepting the letters the Countess wrote to her husband, he sent messengers instead to the Count informing him that, in his absence, his wife was leading a life of gaiety and dissipation. Deeply wounded by his wife's continued silence, the confidence of her husband was at last undermined.

Finally Wlanitz sent word that the Countess had become so shameless in her conduct that she remained away from home for several days at a time, and that her child had at last died of neglect. Maddened by anger and jealousy, Count Sigismond left the Emperor's camp and travelled night and day until he reached the castle. Aloisia was praying in her oratory by an open casement overhanging the precipice, when Sigismond suddenly entered. Startled by the expression on his face, the thought flashed across her mind that her husband had lost his reason, and she stood motionless before him, struck with grief and horror. Mistaking her emotion for guilt, he seized her and threw her from the casement over the precipice. Sigismond then fainted and fell on the floor of the chapel, where for hours he lay in a stupor.

When night came he was suddenly aroused by heavenly harmonies floating through the air outside. Looking through the casement he beheld a beautiful angel floating over the valley, supporting in its arms the forms of his dead wife and child. As the heavenly form passed the window, Sigismond heard a voice saying, "I am a messenger sent from heaven to lead the soul of your sainted wife to the realms of eternal bliss. As you have been betrayed, God in his mercy may forgive you, but He demands the punishment of the traitor by whom you have been deceived." On recovering from the trance Sigismond called his followers together, who, seizing Wlanitz, carried him to the top of the castle, and meted out to him a just retribution by flinging him from the window of the chapel. Sigismond then seized a torch and set fire to his castle, which was soon reduced to a few blackened walls. At daybreak he descended to the village, and putting on the garb of a pilgrim he set out on foot for Rome to obtain pardon of the Pope. On his arrival absolution was granted him by the Holy Father; but, worn out by the privations he had endured on his journey, he sought refuge in a monastery, where he died shortly afterwards.

The village of Engelhaus suffered greatly from a fire in 1885, which destroyed the church and about half the houses in the village.

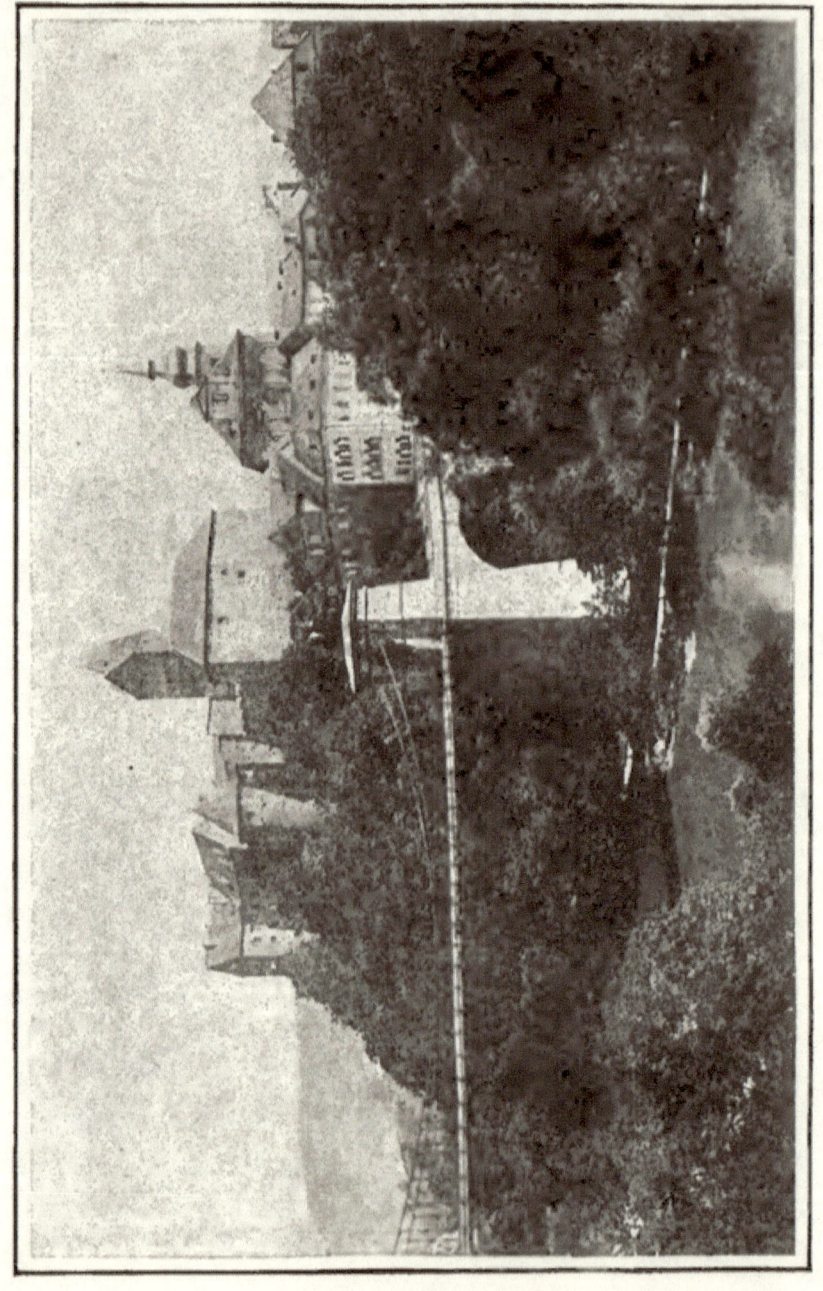

ELBOGEN.

To Elbogen.

Elbogen is from 1¼ to 1½ hour's walk from Carlsbad along the valley of the Eger. It can also be reached by rail, a short branch line connecting the village with the main line to Eger, at the station of *Elbogen Neustattel*. The town, which has a population of about 3000, is picturesquely situated on a rocky peninsula almost surrounded by the Eger, from which the town takes its name of *Elbogen* or "Elbow." Visitors can obtain fair accommodation at the Hotel Zum Weissen Ross, in the market-place, which has a garden and pavilion from which there is a lovely view of the Eger valley, or at the Hotel Scherbaum, near the suspension-bridge. In returning pedestrians can follow the course of the Eger to Hansheilingfels, and have a carriage to meet them at Aich (see. p. 126).

The *Castle of Elbogen*, situated above the village, on a steep granite rock, was founded by the Margraves von Voburg in 870. In 1149 the castle became the property of the German Emperor, Frederick Barbarossa, who received it as a dowry on his marriage with Adelheid, daughter of the Margrave Diebold von Vohburg. In 1434 it came into the possession of the family of the Burgraves Schlick, to whom it belonged for several centuries. In 1725 the castle, along with the town, was almost entirely destroyed by fire, but was afterwards restored. In July 1742 the town and fortress were besieged by the French under General Armitières. The garrison held out for four months, but were at last compelled to surrender through starvation.

From its foundation up to the fourteenth century nothing is known of the history of the castle, as all the records up to that period were destroyed by fire. In 1317 King John of Luxembourg took up his residence for a short time at the castle, accompanied by his wife and infant son, afterwards the Emperor Charles IV. In 1352 Charles IV. granted the citizens of Elbogen a charter, freeing the town from all taxes, under the condition, that whenever he or any of his heirs should visit the town, they should be presented with five pounds of Swabian silver farthings, which were to be handed by the Burgomaster to the sovereign in a wooden beaker. This beaker is still preserved in the Rathhaus, where it may be seen, filled with silver farthings, awaiting the next visit of an Austrian monarch. It was during the visit of the Emperor Charles IV. in 1358 to the Castle of Elbogen that he made his famous hunting expedition to Carlsbad.

During the progress of the Elector Frederick V. and his consort the Princess Elizabeth, daughter of James I. of England, from Heidelberg to Prague to assume the crown of Bohemia, they rested for a night at the Castle of Elbogen, and were magnificently entertained by the Burgrave Schlick at an open-air banquet.

The festivities, however, must have been of a somewhat sober kind, as we are told that after the banquet the Protestant chaplain of the Burgrave preached a sermon of two hours in length to their Majesties on the duties of their high position. The castle is now used as a prison.

The Eger at Elbogen is crossed by a fine suspension-bridge, erected 1833–36 at a cost of 90,000 florins. From the bridge there is a fine view of the river and valley, with the castle above.

In the *Rathhaus* is part of a large meteoric stone which fell at Elbogen, the remaining portion of which weighing 110 pounds, is in the mineralogical museum at Vienna. A model of the stone in its original condition is also to be seen. The stone is locally known as the *Verwünschte Graf*, or "Accursed Count," from the legend that one of the Burgraves of Elbogen had so oppressed the people that they had him cursed with bell, book, and candle. One day shortly afterwards, as he was compelling some of his vassals to undertake some enforced labour, he was struck by a flash of lightning out of a clear sky, and turned into this shapeless mass of stone. In the Rathhaus is also the wooden beaker referred to above.

In the *Deckanal*, or *St. Wencelaus Kirche*, erected in the thirteenth century, and restored after the fire of 1725, is a fine altar-piece by Peter Brandel, representing the murder of St. Wencelaus by his brother

Boleslaus I. before the altar in the Church of Alt Bunzlau in 936.

A *specialité* of Elbogen is the "Elbogener pumpernickel," a kind of gingerbread with a sugar coating. Elbogen has an important porcelain manufactory, over which visitors are shown on application to the office.

To Giesshübl Puchstein.

This is one of the most favourite excursions in the vicinity of Carlsbad. Omnibuses run twice daily. (See page 79.) The drive, which takes about an hour and a half, follows the right bank of the Eger through most picturesque scenery.

Giesshübl, which is rapidly becoming a fashionable watering-place, is beautifully situated on the right bank of the Eger, at the foot of the Buchberg, a rocky and pine-clad hill. The environs are laid out with shady and well-kept paths, and each year the proprietor, Herr Mattoni, adds some new attraction to the place. The general arrangements for the convenience of guests are under the charge of a Cur-committee, who will furnish all information, and, if desired, engage rooms in advance for intending visitors. The number of visitors in 1885 was 18,000. The climate resembles that of Carlsbad.

The springs of Giesshübl have been known for centuries, and were resorted to by the hunters and moun-

GIESSHÜBL-PUCHSTEIN.

taineers in the neighbourhood; but it was only in 1852 that the first spring was enclosed and dedicated to his Majesty Otho, the late King of Greece, who was among the first to visit it. The place, however, owes its rise into prominence to Herr Mattoni, who leased the springs from the proprietor, Baron Neuberg, in 1867, and purchased the Otto Quelle in 1872. Besides conferring a benefit on the public by improving and beautifying this attractive watering-place and its surroundings, he has been eminently successful in a financial way, as the export of Giesshübler water, bottled at the springs, has reached the enormous quantity of 4,000,000 bottles per annum.

The principal building is the *Curhaus*, a handsome stone erection surrounded by gardens and pleasure-grounds. It contains a conversation-room, reading-room, library, and sleeping apartments. Attached to the Curhaus are two '*dependances*.' Near the Curhaus is a *Colonnade*, decorated with a bust of King Otho. The waters of the springs are conducted in pipes both to the Curhaus and to the Colonnade. Opposite the Colonnade is a handsome restaurant with a verandah. On the hill a short distance above Giesshübl is the handsome residence of the proprietor, Herr Mattoni.

The springs are the *Otto Quelle*, or *Giesshübler Sauerbrunn*, *Elizabeth Quelle*, *Franz Josef Quelle*, and the *Löschner Quelle*, which have nearly all the same properties. The following is the analysis of the *Otto Quelle*:—

In 10,000 parts of water—

Silica		0.5941
Chloride of potassium		0.3038
Sulphate ,, ,,		0.3397
Carbonate ,, ,,		0.8240
,, ,, sodium		8.4308
,, ,, lithium		0.0650
,, ,, strontium		0.0230
,, ,, magnesia		1.4004
,, ,, lime		2.3878
Oxide of alumina		0.0290
Oxide of iron		0.0263
,, ,, manganese		0.0099
Organic substances		0.0198
Carbonic acid in combination		5.6004
,, ,, free		23.7396
		43.7936

The waters of Giesshübl are highly charged with carbonic acid gas and are slightly acidulated. They are admirably suited for mixing with wines and spirits, especially with the poorer classes of Austrian and German white wines, as they have the property of almost entirely destroying the acid which is characteristic of these vintages. It is also largely used by itself as a table water. Its effervescence is purely natural, and is therefore free from the injurious results which frequently attend the use of waters which are artificially charged with gas. Giesshübler water has been found to be extremely efficacious in catarrhal affections of the stomach and intestines, jaundice, dyspepsia, and all other complaints caused by a surplus of acid in the system. It has also been found particularly beneficial in cases of catarrhal affection of the respiratory organs. Mixed with warm milk or whey it has a stimulating action on diminished mucous secretion, and at the same time is invigorating and nourishing. In connection with the springs a whey cure has been established.

The spring principally used is the *Otto Quelle*, which is situated on the face of the hill immediately above the Curhaus. Over the spring is a Colonnade supported on fourteen granite pillars, which was inaugurated by King Otho of Greece in 1853. In the Colonnade is a bust of the King, with an inscription commemorating the event. At the spring a new bath-house has lately been erected. The bottling of the waters takes place at this spring, a small railway connecting the bottling establishment with the export warehouse below.

The walks around Giesshübl are charming in their picturesqueness and variety and almost numberless in extent. Well-kept paths have been opened up by the Cur-direction to almost every point of view on the surrounding hills, and on these points little temples, gloriettas and resting-places have been erected, whilst, for feebler visitors, level walks and drives extend both up and down the valley of the Eger.

To Petschau.

The village of Petschau, lying about half-way between Carlsbad and Marienbad (2½ hours' drive), is picturesquely situated overlooking the beautiful valley of the Tepel. In mediæval times the village was of considerable importance, but in 1760 it was almost entirely burned down, and, with the exception of the castle, most of the buildings are now comparatively modern.

The castle, which was erected not later than the eleventh century (as records exist referring to its having been inhabited in 1061), occupies the summit of an eminence overlooking the Tepel. On three sides it is fortified by a wall, and is entered on the south side by a stone bridge, which crosses the old moat, now laid out in gardens. Several of the walls of the castle are of immense thickness. On the left, as we enter, is the ancient round watch-tower, the upper storeys of which were removed in 1623. On the summit of the tower is a platform commanding an extensive panoramic view of the surrounding country. In the interior are a number of large and handsomely decorated apartments, and in the south tower is a Gothic chapel erected in A.D. 1400, the walls of which are decorated with fine frescoes. The view from the windows of the chapel over the valley of the Tepel is exceedingly fine. The castle is still occupied as a residence.

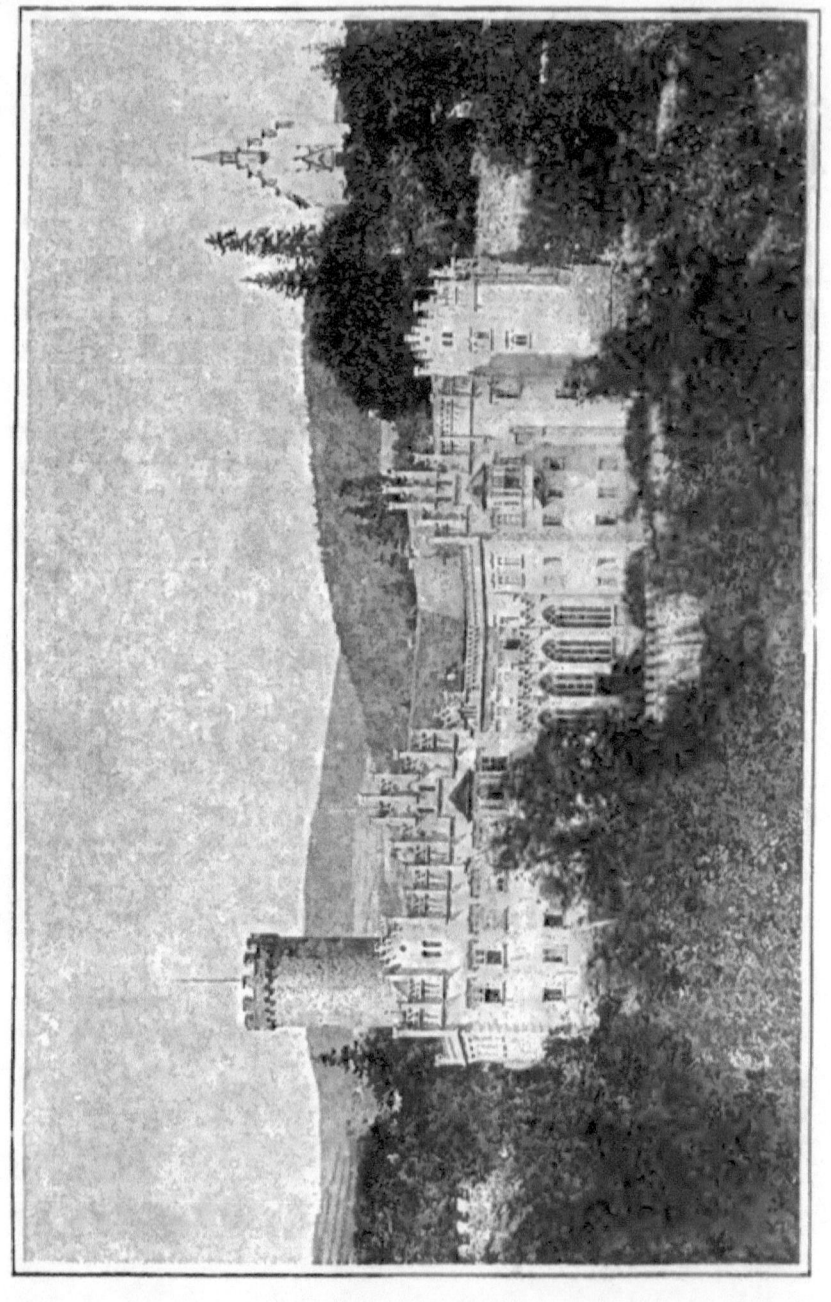

SCHLOSS-HAUENSTEIN.

Visitors are shown over the castle during the absence of the family.

To Schlaggenwald.

The shortest road to the village of Schlaggenwald, passes through Pirkenhammer (see page 126), about $1\frac{1}{2}$ mile beyond which we take the road to Marienbad, and turning off to the left and following the valley of the Tepel, reach Schlaggenwald in about $1\frac{1}{2}$ hour. The village, which is prettily situated, has a porcelain manufactory and a tin and silver mine, which was formerly very productive, but which now hardly pays the expense of working. The parish church is decorated with frescoes executed in 1771 by Dollkopf, who resided for some time at Schlaggenwald. In the Deckanal Kirche is a fine carved altar-piece and a number of tombs of the fourteenth century. Refreshments can be had at the Gasthof zur Krone. Returning we can drive through the picturesque valley of the Zeche, which joins the Eger at Elbogen (see page 137). The drive by Elbogen takes about $2\frac{1}{2}$ hours.

To Schlackenwerth and Hauenstein.

Schlackenwerth can be reached direct by rail, and Hauenstein from the railway station at Hauenstein-Waarte, from which it is about half-an-hour's drive. Carriages are generally found in waiting at Hauenstein-Waarte. The drive from Carlsbad to Schlackenwerth takes about 1½ hour, and to Hauenstein about 2½ hours, the road passing through exceedingly picturesque scenery.

Schlackenwerth is an old town with a château of the Duke of Tuscany, surrounded by a fine park on which is a pavilion with a restaurant. The village has two inns—the Renthaus and Adler.

At *Hauenstein* there is also a small inn, at which visitors can dine, as well as at the restaurant at Hauenstein-Waarte. On the *Eichelberg*, three-quarters of an hour's walk from the village, is the fine modern château of Count J. Buquoi, built in old castellated style. Attached to the château is a beautiful chapel. Surrounding the château and extending over the hill is a magnificent park, intersected by romantic and shady walks. Visitors are not now allowed in the park except by special permission. The summit of the Eichelberg commands one of the most magnificent and extensive views in Germany. In the foreground are the ruined castles of Engelhaus, Himmelstein, Schönburg, and Hauenstein, and below us the fertile valley of the Eger, while in the distance extends the range of the Fichtelbirgen. Of the old castle of Hauenstein only a tower and a fragment of one of the walls remain. In the sixteenth century this old castle was the residence of the Burgrave Heronimus Schlick (see page 34). In the tower the visitor is shown a room in which, during the Thirty Years' War, a Swedish officer was assassinated. The *Himmelstein*, which also commands a lovely view, can be ascended either from Hauenstein or Hauenstein-Waarte.

Pedestrians can return from Hauenstein through *Welchau, Rodisfort,* and *Giesshübl-Puchstein.*

Welchau is a little village prettily situated on the Eger, with a château surrounded by a park in which there are pleasant walks and fine views over the valley. There is a good restaurant, *Zur Linde,* in the village. About one mile beyond Welchau is the village of

Rodisfort, at which there is also a restaurant. Above the village is the *Rodisforterberg,* on the summit of which formerly stood a castle. A legend tells us that in this castle there lived a knight named *Rode,* who was a jovial soul, but always in debt. The patience of his creditors at last becoming exhausted, they proceeded to the castle and swore to hang him over the walls if he did not pay his debts within an hour. The knight having nothing to pay, and having too small a garrison to withstand the siege, did as a good many of the needy fraternity have done since,—he quietly mounted his horse, and leaving the castle by a secret door, made off as fast as he could. Impatient of waiting, his creditors at last broke into the castle, and on inquiring from his vassals where their master was, received the short answer, Rode ist fort — Rode is off — from which the castle and village were afterwards called *Rodisfort.* About half-way up the mountain there is a cave, in which, even in the middle of summer, large icicles are to be seen on the vaulted roof, which show a most charming prismatic colour glancing in the sunbeams which find their way from the entrance. Giesshübl-Puchstein (see page 140) is about 1½ mile beyond Rodisfort.

FALKENAU.

Falkenau is about a half-an-hour's journey by rail on the line to Eger, and two and a half hours' drive from Carlsbad. The carriage road passes through Elbogen (see page 137) and the village of *Altsattel*, near which are the large vitriol, sulphur, and alum works of Herr von Stark. About two miles beyond Altsattel we notice on the bank of the Eger the remains of a landslide which took place in 1832, and which uncovered two extinct volcanoes and partly changed the course of the river.

Falkenau, famous for its hops and its beer, is a busy village of 2500 inhabitants, almost all of whom are employed in the cultivation of the hops and in its large breweries. Beyond its picturesque situation in a hilly but fertile district, its only interest to visitors is the fine castle of Count Nostiz-Rhieneck, which is surrounded by a beautiful park, intersected with lovely walks and drives, and planted with old trees, flowering shrubs, and exotic plants. The castle, which is shown to visitors, contains a fine collection of ancient armour. The best inn is the "Anker."

JOACHIMSTHAL AND THE SONNENWIRBEL, OR KEILBERG.

Joachimsthal, a town of 5500 inhabitants, lies 5½ miles north of Schlackenwerth (see page 146), the road passing through the beautiful valley of the Wistritz. The town was formerly celebrated for its silver-mines, which, although now but little worked, were very productive in the Middle Ages, when they gave employment to over 9000 people. These mines were among the earliest industries of Bohemia. For several centuries after their discovery they were only occasionally rudely mined by the peasants and mountaineers. In 1513 they attracted the notice of the Burgrave, Stephan Schlick, of Carlsbad, who, with the aid of several neighbouring landowners, commenced to work them on a large scale, when they soon became exceedingly productive, yielding between 1516 and 1545 about £1,250,000, an enormous sum at that time. As a German writer naïvely remarks, "There being no Stock Exchange speculations or State lotteries in those days, this was a very nice way of getting money."

Stephan Schlick in 1519 erected a mint here, where he coined the first "Thalers," the name of the coin being a contraction of "Joachimsthaler." These coins had on one side the heads of St. Joachim, and on the other those of King Ludwig of Saxony and the Burgrave Schlick. This old mint is now used as the offices of the mine.

In 1520 Schlick built the castle of Fremdenstein am Berg, near the town, of which only a few scanty ruins remain.

The principal industries of the town are the manufacture of bobbin-lace, woollen yarn, plaited straw, and gloves. In the centre of the town is the inn "Zum Stadt Dresden," where visitors can dine well and cheaply.

About one hour beyond Joachimsthal we come to the village of *Gottesgab* (3300 feet—inn, Grünes Haus), the highest village in Austria, from which we can ascend the *Sonnenwirbel* or *Keilberg*, 4080 feet, the highest point of the Erzgebirge. A carriage road leads to the summit, which commands a magnificent and extensive panoramic view. A tower has been erected on the highest point.

To the north, across the frontier, is the *Fichtelberg* (3985 feet), the highest peak in Saxony. The ascent of the Fichtelberg can be made in about three-quarters of an hour from the village of *Ober-Wiesenthal*, 2½ miles beyond Gottesgab. The summit, on which is a stone tower, commands a most magnificent view, and was formerly an important station in the trigonometrical survey of Central Europe. This excursion requires a long day.

To Kupferberg.

This is one of the pleasantest excursions from Carlsbad. We take the rail to Schlackenwerth, and thence drive past Joachimsthal (see page 148), Gottesgab (see above), and the pretty village of Oberhals to *Kupferberg*, a station on the line from Komatau to Chemitz, where the line reaches its highest point, 2830 feet. The drive takes about four hours.

The view from the little chapel on the summit of the Kupferberg is one of the finest in Austria, and even more extensive than that from the Sonnenwirbel, on a clear day the white hill above Prague and the Drei-Kreuz-Berg above Carlsbad being visible. The return journey can be made by rail

To Fischern, Altrohlau, and Neudeck.

From Carlsbad we take the road crossing the Eger by the Franz Josef's Bridge, and at the station turn to the left, passing through the villages of *Fischern* and *Altrohlau*, both with china manufactories, to *Neudeck*, $3\frac{1}{2}$ hours distant from Carsbad, on the river Rohlau, a busy village, with woollen-mills and tin-factories, and tin and iron mines. Near the village is the handsome new château of Count Asseburg, surrounded by a large park. About a quarter of a mile south of the town are the ruins of an ancient castle, formerly one of the seats of the Barons Schlick. Above the town is the *Kreuzberg*, on the summit of which is a monastery; on the ascent, which winds in zig-zags up the hill, is a *Calvary* with fourteen stone stations of the cross. The hill was purchased by a maiden lady, who expended 27,000 florins in constructing the road and stations, and presented it as a votive offering to the Church. The summit of the hill commands a charming view over the town and surrounding country.

XII.

LONGER EXCURSIONS BY RAIL.

To Eger and Marienbad.

MARIENBAD, though only nineteen miles southward from Carlsbad in a direct line, is about two hours by rail.

An exceedingly pleasant excursion can be made by driving from Carlsbad to Marienbad (about five hours) in a two-horse carriage, and thence returning by rail to Eger.

About an hour after leaving Carlsbad by rail we reach *Eger* (hotels, Wenzel, opposite the station, Erzherzogstephan, in the town), an ancient town with 16,500 inhabitants, situated on the river Eger. It was formerly a free imperial city, and was fortified in 1809. In the *Rathhaus* in the "Ring" the celebrated general, Albert von Wallenstein, the leader of the Imperialists in the Thirty Years' War, was assassinated by an Irishman named Devereux on 25th February 1634. In the rooms in the upper storey, which were those occupied by Wallenstein before his death, there is a museum containing a collection of curiosities and antiquities, among which are the sword, **the writing-table,** and other mementoes of the great general, and the halberd with which he was assassinated. In the museum are also a portrait of Wallenstein and pictures representing his assassination, and the murder of his officers, Illo, Terozky, Kinsky, and Neumann. In the Council Chambers are portraits of the emperors from Leopold I.

Occupying a commanding position on a rock above the river to the north-west of the town are the ruins of the Imperial *Castle*, erected by the Emperor Frederick Barbarossa in 1180, and for several centuries afterwards often occupied by the German emperors. The Castle of Barbarossa was built on the site of a still older fortress, of which the lofty square towers built of blocks of lava, still standing, formed a portion. In the banqueting-room, which adjoins the chapel, the officers of Wallenstein were assassinated a few hours previous to the murder of their general. Since the perpetration of this foul deed the castle has never been inhabited. The terrace above the river commands a fine panoramic view over the town and surrounding country. In the distance rise the three towers of the *Maria-Kulm*, an ancient pilgrimage church, for a long time a haunt of robbers, the bones of whose victims are shown in the chapel.

Fourteen miles beyond Eger we pass the small fortress and spa of *Königswart*, 2250 feet above the level of the sea. The springs, which are chalybeate, are the highest in Germany, and are used both for drinking and bathing. They are recommended in cases of anæmia and incipient consumption. A Curhaus and villas for the reception of visitors have recently been erected.

At Königswart is the château of Prince Metternich, which has been in possession of the family since 1618. The château, which is surrounded by beautifully laid out gardens and pleasure-grounds, contains a collection of coins, minerals, and antiquities, and a gallery of family and historical portraits.

The next station is *Marienbad*. The station is two miles from the town itself. One-horse carriage, 1 fl.; two horses, 1 fl. 80 kr. Omnibus, 40 kr. The best hotels at Marienbad are, "Klinger's," "Neptune," "Hotel Casino," and "Stadt Hamburg." There are also a number of good boarding and lodging houses. The most frequented cafés are the Bellevue, Panorama, Victoria, Miramonte, and Ferdinand's Mühle. Excellent meals and good beer can be had at the Delphin Restaurant. English Church service in the season in the English church erected in 1879, and Presbyterian service in a German Protestant church.

Marienbad is situated in a picturesque valley, about 2000 feet above the level of the sea, above which on three sides rise pine-clad hills. The village is almost entirely modern, having been built since the beginning of the present century. The principal buildings are the Stadthaus, which contains reading and recreation rooms, a large hall used for balls and concerts and other public gatherings, the large military Curhaus erected in 1880, and Roman Catholic, German Protestant, and English churches.

The springs were first brought into public notice in 1870 by the Abbot of the Convent of Tepel. The waters are of much the same character as those of Carlsbad, except that they are of a much lower temperature, ranging from 43° to 50° Fahr., but for bathing they are warmed up to 90°. There are six springs, of which the most used is the Kreuzbrunn, which is a mile distant from the village, the water being conducted in pipes to the Promenade Platz. There are two large bathing-houses, the Alte and the Neue Badhaus, in which are mineral, peat, carbonic acid, and vapour baths. The Marienbad waters, however, are principally used for drinking. The peat found round Marienbad is exceedingly rich in mineral constituents, each cubic foot containing no less than one pound of sulphate of iron. One million bottles of the water from the Kreuzbrunn are annually exported to all parts of the world.

Adjoining the Kreuzbrunn is a beautiful shady avenue 300 yards long, where the visitors promenade from six to eight in the morning while drinking the waters. Close to the spring there is a large brick building, which is used for promenading when the weather is unfavourable. Adjoining this covered promenade is the Bazaar, a double row of shops where Bohemian goods and other *specialités* are sold.

The most abundant of the Marienbad springs is the Ferdinands Brunnen, which is about half a mile distant from the village. The water is carried by pipes to the Promenade Platz, where it flows into a vase of alabaster. The spring which is used for bathing is the Marienquelle; it is highly charged with carbonic acid gas, which keeps the surface of the water in perpetual motion. The quantity of this gas is so great that a light lowered to the surface of the water is immediately extinguished. Gas-baths have been erected at this spring, in which patients are shut up in a box, all except the head, the box being so constructed that the gas is not breathed.

The principal place of resort at Marienbad in fine weather is the *Curgarten*, a prettily laid out pleasure-ground with lawns and parterres, and intersected with pleasant shady walks. Concerts are given in the Promenade Platz from 6 to 7.30 A.M. and from 6 to 7 P.M., and at the Waldquelle from 11.30 A.M. to 12.30 P.M. The season begins about 1st May and lasts till the middle of September.

Marienbad is an exceedingly fashionable spa, and the hotels and boarding-houses are crowded in summer. Rooms should therefore be applied for in advance, in the height of the season. Like Carlsbad, Marienbad is specially attractive from the beauty of its environs, shady walks having been laid out in all directions through the woods and to the best points of view on the hills. The most frequented walk is to the cross on the *Hamelikaberg*, which commands a beautiful view of the valley. Another favourite walk is to the *Mecséry*

Temple, from which there is also a charming and open prospect to the north. The most extensive view, which, however, does not embrace the Wald itself, is to be had from the *Hohendorferhöhe*. A delightful excursion can be made to the *Podhorn* (2750 feet), a mountain of basalt lying to the east, 1½ hour distant from the village. The summit of the mountain commands a most extensive view of the Erzgebirge, Fichtelbirge, and the Bohemian forest. A longer, but also a most charming excursion can be made to the wealthy Abbey of Tepel, to which the spring at Marienbad belongs. The Abbey, which lies nine miles east of Marienbad, contains an extensive library and a Zoological and Geological Museum. There are also various other objects of interest which are shown to visitors.

To Franzensbad.

Franzensbad, which lies west of Carlsbad, is reached in about 2½ hours by railway. The best hotels are the Adler, Post, Hubner, British Hotel, Müller's Hotel, the Erzherzogin Gisela, and the Kaiser von Oesterreich. Restaurants at the Cursaal, Railway Station, Weilburg, Brandenburg Thor, Prince of Wales, the latter with gardens.

The springs of Franzensbad, which are situated on a level plain 1570 feet above the sea, are principally frequented by ladies, the iron spring and peat baths being highly recommended for female complaints. The annual number of visitors is about 10,000, only a small proportion of whom belong to the male sex. The climate is bracing, but the changes in temperature are often very sudden and somewhat trying. About 200 houses have been erected at this spa, almost all of which are devoted to the accommodation of visitors.

The principal building is the *Cursaal*, a large structure containing reading and conversation rooms, restaurant, and a large concert salon 150 feet long and 52 feet wide. For shelter in unfavourable weather there are two colonnades, one of wood lined with shops, which extends from the Franzensquelle to the Cursaal, and another of brick, 220 yards in length, has been erected at the Salzquelle.

In fine weather the visitors promenade in a large and beautifully laid out park, which extends from the city to the railway station. In the park there is a bronze statue of Francis I., the founder of the baths. There are several large bathing establishments at the spa, about one-half of the baths being mineral, and the remainder peat baths, which are greatly used. The Franzensbad peat, like that of Marienbad, is extremely rich in sulphate of iron. The springs, which are cold (50° Fahr.), are ferruginous and are highly tonic, the principal ingredients being iron, carbonic acid, soda, and Glauber salts. The principal spring is the *Franzensquelle*, where most of the visitors assemble from 4.30 to 6.30 P.M. to drink the waters and listen to the orchestra. Life at Franzensbad, however, is dull at its best, as the majority of the patients are feeble and suffering, and the absence of the male sex gives a somewhat one-sided character to the conversation and amusements.

To Teplitz.

Teplitz, next to Carlsbad the most celebrated and the most frequented of the Austrian watering-places, lies west from Carlsbad about three hours' distance by rail. The hotels are the Stadt London, Post, Altes-Rathhaus, König von Preussen, and Schwartz's Ross; at Schönau, the Neptun. The best and most frequented restaurants and cafés are at the Cursaal, in the Stephan's Platz, and the Garten Salon, in the Schlossgarten; at both of these *table d'hôte* is served during the season. There are also restaurants at the hotels. Excellent confectionery at Müller's in the Bäder Platz and Zimma in the Curgarten. English Church service is held during the season. A new Theatre has been erected in the Curgarten, at which performances are given daily. Concerts are given in the Curgarten daily from 6.30 to 8 A.M., in the Schlossgarten from 11 A.M. to 1 P.M. In the evening concerts are given alternately in the Cur-garten and the Schlossgarten. Balls are held in the Garten salon every Saturday evening from 8 to 12 P.M.

Teplitz, which takes its name from a Slavonic word signifying "warm bath," lies in the broad and fertile valley of the Bela, 725 feet above the sea-level. It is an ancient town with 16,000 inhabitants, and is one of the oldest watering-places in Europe, the spring having been known as early as the eighth century. The number of visitors is about 12,000 annually.

The life at Teplitz is a great contrast to that of most of the other watering-places in the north of Austria, as it is a quiet and comparatively cheap place; but, nevertheless, it is by no means dull, while, with its splendid gardens and beautiful environs, it even outrivals its gayer sisters of Carlsbad and Marienbad. The season lasts from May till September, but the baths are open the whole year.

The springs, which are saline-alkaline, have a temperature of 86° to 118° Fahr., and are used both for drinking and bathing. They have a stimulating and exciting effect, and are considered exceedingly beneficial in cases of rheumatism, gout, paralysis, and nervous disorders.

As in Carlsbad, the visitors at Teplitz assemble to take the waters and promenade at the Trinkhalle in the Curgarten between 6 and 8 A.M. Another favourite promenade is the grounds of the *Château of Prince Clary*, where the visitors assemble from 11 A.M. to 1 P.M. to listen to the concerts which are given between these hours. In the grounds, which are beautifully laid out, are a café restaurant and a dairy. On the south-east side of the Curgarten, in the Stephan's Platz, are the *Cursalon*, with reading and conversation rooms, restaurant, and café, and the *Kaiserbad*, a magnificent structure, fitted up with bath-rooms and elegantly furnished apartments. On the opposite side of the Garten is the new Theatre, a handsome building of Renaissance architecture.

The favourite walks are to the *Königshöhe* (820 ft.), an eminence lying immediately to the south of the town, on which is the *Schlackenberg*, a curious roccoco erection of sandstone and glazed bricks. In the building is a restaurant, and from the tower (camera obscura 15 kr.) there is a fine panoramic view of the town and the Bela valley. Charming views can also be obtained from the Belvidere restaurant and from the café Villa Bellavista.

A short distance from the Curgarten, on the road to the Schlackenberg, is a monument erected in honour of Frederick William III. of Prussia in 1841, by "Grateful Teplitz," to commemorate the visits of the emperor to the baths.

To the east side of the town lies the suburb of *Schönau*, which was formerly a separate village, but is now united to Teplitz by terraces of new houses. At Schönau there are also extensive bath-houses and ample accommodation for visitors.

Between Teplitz and Schönau is a small hill, the *Mont de Ligne*, on the summit of which is a restaurant and a belvidere, the latter commanding a fine panoramic view of the town and its environs.

East of Schönau is the *Schlossberg* (1280 feet), which can be ascended in about half an hour. On the summit are the ruins of an ancient castle destroyed by the Imperialist troops in A.D 1655 during the Thirty Years' War.

A pleasant excursion from Teplitz can be made to the baths of *Eichwald*, 1378 feet above the level of the sea, which is delightfully situated amid beautiful wooded scenery, three miles to the north-west. An omnibus runs between Teplitz and Eichwald several times daily.

Another favourite excursion can be made to the *Mileschauer* or *Donnersberg*, a hill 2740 feet in height, lying about ten miles to the south-east. The summit, on which there is an inn, commands one of the most extensive and picturesque views in Bohemia. Visitors take the stage or a carriage (two hours) from Teplitz to Pilkau, from which it is about an hour's walk to the summit.

XIII.

SHOOTING AND FISHING.

VERY fair shooting and fishing can be enjoyed by visitors in the neighbourhood of Carlsbad. For shooting, a licence ("waffenpass"), price 1 fl., must be obtained from the Burgomaster, and leave must also be obtained from the shooting society. Shooting begins on the 1st August, and ends on the 31st January; the best time for winged game being August and the beginning of September, and for ground game and deer the late autumn and winter months. Cartridges to fit English guns can be obtained from Rosenfeldt's Wisen Lowen, Markt Platz, and A. Epstein, Goldener Lowen, opposite the Curhaus. The game in the neighbourhood of Carlsbad consists of partridge (rebbahn), blackcock (birkhahn), hares (hasen), and deer (reh), also a very few wild boar.

The fish in the streams near Carlsbad are trout (forellen), best season May and June, which run from 4 to 6 to the pound, with an occasional half-pounder or even larger, pike, barm, rothauge—very game fish with red eyes, which run from 3 to 6 pounds—and weissfisch (white fish), which average from 1 to 3 pounds.

Visitors are permitted to fish in the Eger provided they are accompanied by one of the fishermen of the Fischerei-Verein, who expects a small honorarium. All fish caught must be given up to the society or paid for at the market price. For fishing in the Eger tickets are issued by the Fischerei-Verein, price 3 florins per month. Fish caught can be kept by the angler.

For trout the best baits are artificial flies, worms, and grasshoppers. The small boys about Carlsbad will gladly collect a packet of either of the latter for visitors. Flies can be obtained at Rosenfeldt's and Epstein's. Barm and rothauge are taken in the same way as trout. For weissfisch, which in the summer months are very plentiful and take freely, the best bait is whole cherries, either black or red. These fish lie in the necks of the pools, which should be baited the previous day by throwing in quantities of cherries. They take most freely in the mornings and evenings.

The best rivers are the Tepel, the Petschau, the Eger (no trout), the Neudeck, and the Weissbach. In the district round Carlsbad there are a number of deep ditches which contain large carp. They give, however, very little sport.

XIV.

THE EXPORTATION AND PRODUCTS OF THE CARLSBAD SPRINGS.

THE exportation of the Carlsbad water is comparatively a new industry, the first water for export having been bottled in 1842. For a long time it was supposed that the waters lost their efficacy after they became cold. This prejudice was removed by Dr. Hlawacek, who proved incontestably that after being heated again to their normal temperature they still retained most of their medicinal properties. It is impossible, however, to contend that the exported waters are of equal efficacy to those drunk at the springs, not only from the possible escape of their most volatile constituents, but from the absence of the salutary effect of the change of air and regular mode of life, which are in themselves most valuable aids to recovery. Besides this, their beneficial influence is often greatly increased by bathing in the same water, which of course is only possible at Carlsbad itself.

166   EXPORTATION AND PRODUCTS OF THE SPRINGS.

Nevertheless the exported waters are often of value in cases of sudden emergency, or when the patient finds it impossible to visit the springs; they are also of great use in completing the cure after the visit is ended. The waters best suited for exportation are those of the cooler springs, as they contain the greatest amount of carbonic acid gas, those most used for the purpose, therefore, being the Marktbrunn, Schlossbrunn, and Mühlbrunn.

The bottles are packed in cases and sold in Carlsbad at the following prices, cases included:—

		fl.
Case of 50 bottles	. . . .	13
,, 30 ,,	. . . .	9
,, 12 ,,	. . . .	12

Sprudel Salt was first prepared by Dr. Berger in 1708, though his experiments were only tentative. In 1732 Dr. Borrias discovered a method of obtaining the salt in sufficient quantities for export by evaporating the water and crystallising the deposit. This process he made over to Dr. Richter, who obtained from the Emperor Charles VI. the right to manufacture the salt. At first the townspeople objected strongly to the preparation and sale of the salt, fearing that it would do away with the necessity of visitors coming to Carlsbad. This absurd prejudice at last became so strong that the manufacture of the salt was stopped for several years, and it was only allowed to be given to patients actually resident at Carlsbad.

In 1764 Dr. David Becker discovered a new process of preparing the salt by using the natural heat of the Sprudel itself as the means of evaporation.

By this method a much larger quantity of the salts was able to be produced, and its price was greatly reduced. Shortly after this a Government act was passed permitting the exportation of the salt, and the townspeople, finding that this had rather the effect of attracting the attention of the public to the springs than of keeping visitors away, soon got rid of their prejudices.

The demand for the salt rapidly increased, until in 1813 it was found necessary to erect a building for its manufacture, connected by pipes with the Sprudel. In 1863 the Government leased the manufacture of the salt to Herr Mattoni, who built a stone factory near the Ferdinand's Brücke. In 1877 Herr Mattoni's contract expired, and the factory was let to Herr L. Schottloender for ten years, at an annual rent of 70,000 florins. The constantly increasing demand for the salt has necessitated the extension of the factory, till it is now one of the largest and most completely appointed in Europe.

In 1880 the Carlsbad Town Council commissioned the celebrated analyist, Dr. Ernest Ludwig of Vienna, to undertake experiments with the view of obtaining a salt from the springs which, when dissolved, should more nearly resemble the natural mineral water than the Sprudel Salt. He succeeded in obtaining a preparation which he named *Natural Carlsbad Salt*, and which contains all the properties of the springs themselves. It has also the advantage of being less liable to evaporation when exported. The Natural Salts, which are packed in bottles of 100 and 200 grammes ($\frac{1}{5}$ and $\frac{2}{5}$ lb.) with green labels, have now almost superseded the Sprudel Salt.

The salt is used either dissolved in the mineral water to increase its cathartic action, the dose being one to two drachms to a tumbler of the water, or by dissolving a small teaspoonful in half a tumbler of hot water, or better still, of Giesshübl, Krondorf, or soda water.

The Natural Carlsbad Salt is a most valuable mild cathartic, as it operates quickly and without pain. It has also the advantage that the dose does not require to be increased after a time as with most other cathartics, nor does constipation follow after its use is discontinued. The salt should be taken in the morning before breakfast.

The Natural Carlsbad Salts are also made into pastilles, which are taken for acidity, heartburn, and flatulency. Two to four pastilles should be taken two to three times daily, preferably about half an hour after meals.

The salt contains in 100 parts—

	Per cent.
Carbonate of lithium	0.39
Bicarbonate of soda	35.95
Sulphate of potash	3.25
Sulphate of soda	42.03
Chloride of soda	18.16
Fluoride of soda	.09
	99.87

The *Sprudel Soap* is prepared from the lye, or first deposit of the Sprudel water, after the crystallised salts have been extracted. This lye contains about fourteen cent. of mineral constituents.

This chemical compound is purified from all traces of Glaubers' salt, and by the addition of lime is turned into caustic lye, from which the soap is manufactured by the ordinary process. The soap, which possesses considerable healing power, is beneficial in cases of chronic diseases of the skin, and is used in both plain and mineral water baths. It is also used for poulticing cold abscesses and boils, and for making a soap embrocation.

Part II.

MEDICAL TREATISE.

I.

ACTION OF THE WATERS.

BESIDES the stimulating properties common to most mineral waters, those of Carlsbad possess three special properties of their own.

(1.) By their high temperature they accelerate the absorption, stimulate the circulation of the blood, produce perspiration, and act as a sedative upon the nervous system.

(2.) The carbonic acid gas which they contain augments the secretion of gastric juice, stimulates the appetite and the digestion, calms the gastric nerves, and strengthens the peristaltic movements of the stomach and intestinal tract.

(3.) Their use results in a specific action, viz., a chemical modification in the system by the *introduction of the alkaline salts*, the *sulphates and carbonates of soda*, and the *chloride of sodium*. They are *anti-acid* par excellence, and the *sulphate of soda* is a mild *laxative*. Alkalies among other things have been proved to be indispensable to the phenomena of endosmosis, combustion, digestion, and secretion;

they contribute to maintain the blood in the degree of viscosity necessary to keep it fitted for endosmosis, exosmosis, the different compositions and decompositions which constitute existence. They render the saccharine and amylaceous matters, introduced by alimentation, capable of combining with the oxygen and assisting in the functions of respiration and calorification. They cause the elements of the bile to become fluid, prevent them from thickening or forming calculi, maintain the intestinal digestion, facilitate the secretions, and thus influence all the acts of nutrition and assimilation. The Carlsbad waters, in rendering the blood more alkaline, cause it to lose a part of its coagulatory properties; they attack the albumen and the fibrine, and bring about promptly the dissolution of these substances. If the blood, having become more fluid, moves with more liberty in its channels, and if, besides, it possesses the property of dissolving the two principal elements which form the basis of most chronic congestions, a near approach has been attained to a knowledge of the mechanism by which the Carlsbad waters are dissolvent, resolutive, antiplastic, and deobstruent. It is, therefore, of extreme importance to pay particular attention to the double action, tonic and chemical, of those waters when using them for the treatment of different diseases.

From their exciting and tonic properties their use is not advisable in acute inflammatory disorders, in cases in which chronic inflammations have a tendency to assume an acute form, and in those in which the viscera are subject to serious disorganisation, the progress of which is generally aggravated by anything that accelerates the circulation. On the other hand, they are beneficial in chronic affections, if it is required to give a particular stimulus to the organs, to promote the circulation, excite the secretions, or regulate nutrition and assimilation.

By their chemical properties they are suitable in all cases of congestion, obstruction of the viscera, as *catarrh of the stomach, catarrh of the bowels, biliary and urinary calculi, disorders of the liver, gravel, catarrh of the bladder, gout, rheumatism,* and *diabetes*. Practical observation shows that they produce *beneficial modifications in lymphatic or scrofulous constitutions, as well as in albuminuria*. But they should be employed with great caution and prudence by cachectic, consumptive, or emaciated patients, who, though they sometimes derive advantage from their stimulating virtues, have to fear, on the other hand, an aggravation of their condition.

The Carlsbad springs present, in their medical aspect, differences much more important than might be supposed from their chemical analysis. By their stimulating and at the same time alterative properties the same springs often present the greatest contrasts. According to the constitution of the persons and the nature of the disease they produce calm or excitement, sleep or wakefulness, diarrhœa or constipation; they soothe or increase certain pains, strengthen or weaken, fatten or reduce.

The first sensation on taking the waters is decidedly pleasant. After a short use of them a genial warmth spreads itself over the body, and a feeling of comfort and lightness is experienced. In some cases, after the first week, the pains or symptoms from which the patient is suffering are greatly increased (called the *crisis*), but this need not in the least degree excite fear or apprehension. In a few days the unpleasantness passes away, and then rapid improvement takes place. The complexion gradually clears day by day, and by the end of the course it assumes a natural and healthy tinge.

II.

USE OF THE MINERAL WATERS AT CARLSBAD.

FOR the right use of the waters it is very necessary that a correct diagnosis of each case should be formed. For this reason the invalid should always seek the advice of a physician who has made a special study of the diseases upon which the Carlsbad waters are supposed to exercise a salutary influence. The following explanation, therefore, of the treatment is only intended to induce the patient to follow the directions of the physician more intelligently.

The usual regime is, to commence with, from three half to three whole tumblers of the special spring prescribed by the medical attendant, taken at intervals of a quarter of an hour, and increasing gradually to three, four, five, and six tumblers.

The waters are taken in the morning as a rule, the usual hours being from 6 to 8 A.M., except in the case of delicate invalids, who may be permitted to breakfast lightly beforehand if necessary, and even to use the waters at home.

The patient should rise about 6 A.M., so as to reach the spring about 6.30 A.M. To go early to the spring has many advantages, as it not only avoids loss of time, and consequent hurry, a serious consideration for patients subject to congestion in the head and perspiration; but at that time, the stomach being empty, the water will be more easily absorbed. Here at the different springs are to be met people of all classes and from every country—crowned heads and princes of royal blood, members of the English aristocracy, Americans, French, Germans, Russians, Swedes, Turks, &c. Ailments of almost every form are likewise represented, and it is a most interesting sight to watch the daily improvement in health and spirits of many who had probably considered their cases hopeless. There is a covered colonnade at each of the principal springs, which can be used in wet weather, and an excellent band plays every morning from 6 to 8, thereby assisting the cure, by diverting the mind and enlivening the spirits. Between the times of drinking the waters the patient should promenade, as far as his strength or the complaint from which he suffers will allow, and after the last draught should, if possible, take a walk of an hour's duration.

Exercise facilitates the absorption of the waters, and is also necessary to the re-establishment of health. After the walk breakfast should be taken.

III.

EXTERNAL USE OF THE MINERAL WATER.

ALTHOUGH drinking the waters at Carlsbad constitutes the principal means of cure, experience and observation teach us that by bathing their effects are considerably increased. To assist the operation of the waters, mineral, mud, iron, vapour, or douche baths are prescribed, and for this purpose there are several bathing establishments fitted up with every requisite. The special form of baths, their temperature, the frequency with which they should be taken, and the time which the patient should remain in them, must depend upon their special case and on the advice of their medical attendant.

The Sprudel Water is conducted in long iron pipes to the *Curhaus*, to the *Stadthaus*, and to the *Neubad*, where it is cooled to the requisite degree.

The *peat bath* consists of *black peat*. This peat is rich in mineral constituents. It is first pulverised, then screened and freed from accidental impurities, mixed with the hot Sprudel Water, or, as in the Neubad, heated by steam when the bath is ordered. The usual temperature of the Sprudel bath ranges from 80° Fahr. to 96° Fahr.; of the peat bath, from 96° Fahr. to 100° Fahr.; of the vapour bath, from 100° Fahr. to 130° Fahr. The baths are taken either in the morning when fasting, after drinking the mineral water, or about two hours after breakfast, generally between 11 and 1 o'clock in the forenoon. During the bath any affected parts, such as the region of the spleen and liver or inflamed or stiffened joints, should be subjected to gentle friction.

Before taking the bath all excitement or fatigue, or anything that is liable to accelerate the circulation of the blood, or produce palpitation of the heart or congestion of the brain, must be carefully avoided. A bath must never be taken on a full stomach, and three hours at least should be allowed to elapse after a meal. Strong persons may take their bath in the morning after drinking the waters and before breakfast, but weak patients should not bathe till after having had a meal.

The nature of the bath, the number necessary to be taken, and the duration of the bath must always be determined by the physician, as he has in prescribing to take into consideration the nature of the disease, the age and constitution of the patient, and the chemical composition of the water or peat.

It very often occurs at Carlsbad that patients after having taken a number of mineral or peat baths get an eruption on the skin, sometimes itching, called the "badfriesel" or "bath-rush." This eruption, however, need occasion no alarm, as it is only due to the action on the skin of the salt in the water or peats. The eruption entirely disappears when the baths are stopped for two or three days.

As the greater number of patients suffering from chronic rheumatism, gout, or skin eruptions are liable to a profuse perspiration after taking the baths, they should always be provided with warm clothing. In warm weather they may take a short walk after the bath, but in damp or cold weather they should immediately return home and rest for a short time.

Patients who are in the slightest degree subject to congestion of the brain should, especially if they take peat baths, keep a cold wet towel on their heads as long as they remain in the bath, and they should also be careful to have an attendant at hand to change the towels as they become warm.

IV.

DIETETICS DURING THE USE OF THE WATERS.

NOT less important than drinking the waters and taking the baths is the proper management of the patient's regimen. It is of the most vital importance that the patient at Carlsbad should lead a *regular life;* retire early, rise early, eat and drink moderately, and always at the same hour of the day. He should be the whole day, if possible, in the open air, and should take constant but moderate exercise, but be most careful to avoid all fatigue or exhaustion. Above all, he should keep his mind free from worry about business affairs, or any other matters requiring anxious thought, as the mind requires rest as well as the body.

Bathing and drinking the waters cannot effect a cure if the diet and method of life, and even the amusements, are not regulated by the rules of the special case. Especially the diet and the amount of exercise has to be prescribed by the medical attendant.

The *diet* should be always nourishing but simple. The desire for food is generally increased; but as the main object of the use of the waters is restoration to health, reason must regulate the diet. It is very important that there should be a considerable interval between each meal. Experience proves that the stomach requires from four to five hours to digest the quantity of food eaten at a moderate meal, and after this process the stomach remains for almost an hour in an abnormal condition, which may be compared to a slight catarrh. It is only after the lapse of five to six hours that the stomach resumes its ordinary healthy condition. Three meals during the day are generally sufficient.

The common custom in Carlsbad is as follows:— After having drunk the requisite number of cups of mineral water early in the morning, a good hour's walk is prescribed before taking *breakfast*, between 8 and 9 o'clock. This meal consists of coffee or tea with milk, a moderate quantity of toast or roll (without butter), and a couple of eggs or a small quantity of cold meat. Butter, fat, or grease of any kind is expressly forbidden.

The greater number of visitors to Carlsbad take their breakfast in the open air. In the gardens and at the restaurants the most delicious coffee and tea and excellent Vienna rolls (Semmel & Kipfel) are served at little tables under verandahs and beneath the shade of the trees. Having rested a while after breakfast, another short walk should be taken before bathing-time, which is generally between 10 and 11 A.M. After the bath a rest should be taken before dinner.

At Carlsbad *table d'hôte* dinners are not customary, as nearly all of the patients have to follow a certain regimen prescribed by their physician. Besides this, no dishes at the hotels or restaurants which are unsuitable for patients taking the mineral waters (so-called "curgemäss" or "against the cure rules") are allowed to be put on the bills of fare.

Dinner is usually taken between the hours of one and two. It consists of three to four dishes, as soup (not always), fish, roast beef, roast veal, or roast chicken; and green vegetables, such as spinach, cauliflower, asparagus, French beans, or green peas, &c., and stewed fruits (*compôte*). The patients should be careful not to overload the stomach; any objectionable or injurious food, such as raw fruits, ices, sour or too sweet dishes, are to be avoided. Stimulants of good quality, such as claret, hock, pilsener beer, when taken in *moderation*, in no way diminish the effects of the mineral waters; they often, indeed, serve as a stimulant to the system. But, at the same time, spirits, such as brandy and whisky, must be strictly avoided, as they may lead to the most serious consequences. A short rest after dinner (but no sleep), and then a stroll through the woods or a walk to some of the pleasure-gardens outside the town, where there is music, brings the time up to 6 P.M., at which hour tea with milk and eggs, or a chop, or cold meat, is usually taken, and by 9 or 10 o'clock most people retire to bed, rising up refreshed the next morning to go through precisely the same course as on the preceding day.

Over-fatigue or unnecessary exertion is to be particularly avoided; but, at the same time, as fresh air greatly assists the cure, patients are advised to be out as much as possible so long as the weather admits of it, taking especial care, however, not to get chilled.

The climate of Carlsbad, like that of most mountainous districts, is liable to sudden changes, especially during the morning and evenings; and as patients have to be the greater part of the day out of doors taking exercise, and so liable to perspire freely, they should always wear flannel undershirts and be provided with a shawl or an overcoat.

Smoking is to be restricted within the narrowest limits.

Sleeping during the day is generally unadvisable. Weak persons, however, who sleep badly during the night may sleep for about half an hour before dinner.

Occupation.—During the use of the waters the patient ought to avoid all kinds of business. The beneficial effect of the waters will be much assisted if the patient's mind be at rest during his stay at our watering-place, where he will find the most beautiful walks and drives among the charming and picturesque woods and mountains. Other patients need and find pleasant society and cheerful company at Carlsbad. The excellent bands of music and the famous classical concerts also contribute much to the general enjoyment. To the artist and lover of scenery Carlsbad presents numberless charms; and the views to be seen from the *Aberg*, the *Hirschensprung*, the *Panorama*, and the *Dreikreuzberg* are magnificent, and should on no account remain unvisited. A few miles distant are *Hammer*, *Hansheiling* and *Giesshübl*. Hansheiling is a lovely spot in the valley of the Eger, and at Giesshübl there is a natural spring from which the water issues forth as cold as ice and effervescing like soda water.

V.

GENERAL INDICATIONS FOR THE USE OF CARLSBAD WATER.

CASES IN WHICH THE WATERS ARE DECIDEDLY INDICATED, AND THOSE IN WHICH THEY ARE CONTRA-INDICATED.

CHRONIC conditions of every form of abdominal disease are the most likely to be benefited by the water. They are not in all cases completely cured, but it very rarely happens that they are not modified in their worst symptoms. Most of our patients are affected with *Plethora abdominalis*, arising from too substantial and abundant nourishment, combined with a sedentary life, where chylification exceeds the ordinary want of nature. The blood is therefore overloaded with the final results of the digestion, and all the secretions are disturbed. The excretory organs are found incapable of eliminating the superfluous matters, and this being retained, morbid products came to be developed. The quantity as well as the quality of the blood and of the other fluids being thus injuriously altered, many chronic diseases arise, such as indigestion, constipation, gout, piles, gallstones, renal calculi, gravel, gouty eczema, &c. &c. In these complaints the waters are very efficacious on account of their action on the bowels, on the urinary organs, and on the skin, which tends to diminish the amount of the solid constituents of the blood and otherwise to restore it to its normal condition.

Special Indications.

1. *Dyspepsia.* At least two-thirds of the patients to be met with at Carlsbad go there in order to obtain from the waters relief from the varied forms of indigestion. They frequently complain that they have little or no appetite. After eating they feel heaviness and pain in the epigastrium, flatulence, acidity, headache, weakness, and depression. When the dyspepsia is simple and idiopathic it is generally cured in a complete and easy manner by the use of the Carlsbad waters.

But dyspepsia depends also very frequently on chronic or constitutional affections, and manifests itself as a secondary symptom of some predominant disease, such as chronic catarrh of the stomach, ulcer of the stomach, gout, &c. Even in these cases patients have often obtained the most favourable results, as the thermal treatment has a very beneficial influence on those chronic and constitutional maladies.

It happens very often with a dyspeptic patient, as one of the consequences of the slowness of the digestion, that the local nervous system becomes excited to such a point as to give rise to neuralgic symptoms. This painful neurosis of the stomach, or *gastralgia*, manifests itself under several forms.

2. The typical form is the attack of *gastralgia* or cramp in the stomach—cramps, both violent and lasting from half an hour to several hours. It begins with headache, pain in the epigastrium and back, accompanied with dyspnœa and vomiting, and finishing with exhaustion. There are a certain number of cases in which we find combined both the symptoms of gastralgia and dyspepsia, namely, *gastralgic dyspepsia* or *dyspeptic gastralgia*, according to which of those forms predominates.

Gastralgia and dyspepsia, however distinct they may be from each other, may therefore meet on the same ground, and thus necessitate those therapeutic measures which apply to both. Carlsbad waters produce in both cases the most satisfactory results. Another most disagreeable consequence of *chronic catarrh of the stomach* is

3. *The dilatation of the stomach.* The slightest pressure on a greatly distended stomach easily produces a *visible undulation* and *gurgling noise*, accompanied by dyspepsia, gastralgia, flatulency, frequent eructations of sour liquid and air, palpitation of the heart, vomiting, dyspnœa, and general exhaustion. This complaint, when far advanced, is seldom completely cured, but it can decidedly be very much improved by washing

out the stomach with Carlsbad water, introduced and withdrawn through a stomach tube and funnel like a siphon.

Besides this innocent, painless, and most efficacious treatment *massage* and *electricity* may be applied to the dilated stomach.

4. *Chronic catarrh of the bowels, chronic diarrhœa*, as well as *chronic constipation*, and their consequences, all being different species of the same affection, find generally a quick and radical remedy in the Carlsbad waters.

5. *Colic*, a neuralgia of the intestinal nerves, and perhaps also of the ramifications of the mesenteric plexus, characterised by constringent, wandering, or fixed pains in the umbilical region and the colon, is often cured at Carlsbad. Also the *Colica saturnina* (Colic of Devonshire), the so-called lead poisoning, finds a remedy in the Carlsbad waters.

The Carlsbad waters have no anthelmintic or worm-destroying action, properly speaking, notwithstanding that *Ascarides lumbricoïdes* and *oxyuris vermicularis*, and even great lengths of *tapeworm* are often expelled by them; they, however, have a great influence in destroying the tendency to the formation of worms.

6. *Diseases of the liver and biliary ducts* are also treated with most successful results at the hot alkaline springs of Carlsbad, especially *enlargements of the liver* of various kinds, occasioned principally by *accumulation of fat* or by *congestion*. The waters are, however, of

little or no use if the enlargement of the liver is caused by cancer or by encysted echinococcus.

Cirrhosis of the liver can only be benefited in its earlier stages. In *nearly all cases of jaundice* where the discharge of the bile into the intestine is prevented, either by gastric catarrh having extended into the duodenum and biliary ducts or by chronic inflammation in the liver, or when it is prevented by any other interruption of the flow of the bile, such as some strong nervous perturbation or gallstones, Carlsbad waters are particularly efficacious.

7. *Gallstones* and *hepatic colics* are diseases in which the favourable effects of the Carlsbad springs may be looked for with the greatest certainty. The fact is, that under the influence of the thermal treatment the expulsion of gallstones and gravel is often singularly facilitated, sometimes without pain, but more frequently with the most painful colics, which may occur at Carlsbad or immediately after the thermal treatment. Such attacks of violent colic occurring either during or after the use of the Carlsbad waters indicate invariably a considerable amelioration of the disease, if not its entire disappearance.

Our alkaline waters not only facilitate the expulsion of smaller concretions through the biliary ducts into the duodenum, but also seem to act upon the bile, so as to do away either temporarily or altogether with tendency to this species of lithiasis or forming of gallstones. Carlsbad is a sure remedy also for *polycholia*, the excessive secretion of bile, generally the consequence of an hereditary bilious constitution, of a residence in tropical climates, of too luxurious and heating food, or of the abuse of mercury and the iodides.

Also the functional derangements of the spleen, especially enlargement of that organ as a consequence of malaria and intermittent and typhoid fever, are generally not only improved but completely cured in Carlsbad.

8. Our waters are also specially useful in dissolving and expelling *gravel* and *small calculi of the kidneys and bladder*. Patients suffering from gravel or calculi soon feel in Carlsbad a great relief from their complaint. The urine becomes alkaline. Being secreted more abundantly and without pain, it dissolves and carries off the glairy and purulent matters resulting from irritation of the mucous membrane, soon ceases to be thick and fœtid, and becomes limpid; while at the same time *hæmaturia* or blood in the urine, *nephritic* or kidney *colics*, pain in the kidneys and bladder, and the disorders caused by the presence of calculi are diminished and removed. Sleep, appetite, and strength revive, and patients who on arriving could scarcely stand are able in a few days to take salutary exercise. It has been proved by practical tests that the Carlsbad springs, being strongly charged with bicarbonate of soda, dissolve and disintegrate the different ingredients of the calculi, and assist in their natural expulsion from the bladder. The waters dissolve the animal matter, and as a consequence separate the saline parts, which,

deprived of their cement, are deposited in small scales and expelled with the urine. In this manner the waters may act on the *phosphatic calculi,* especially on those of *ammoniacal-magnesian-phosphate,* as well as on the calculi of *uric acid.*

The effect of the waters is indeed not only to neutralise the uric diathesis, and for the time to prevent it from manifesting itself, but also to modify the organic causes of its production, by rendering the urine alkaline before its arrival in the kidneys and bladder. Also the efficacy of our alkaline springs is incontestably evident in cases where the urine is neutral or alkaline, muddy, fœtid, or discoloured, containing phosphatic (white) gravel deposits and calculi of phosphate of lime, or of ammoniac-magnesia-phosphate, or of a mixture of this latter with phosphate of lime, as well as in cases of non-ammoniac-phosphatic gravel and calculi. By the introduction of a large quantity of bicarbonate of soda into the system they modify the pathological state of the mucous membrane of the bladder and liquefy the thickened mucus. They also act on the composition of the blood, by preventing the formation of uric acid or neutral phosphates; thus they change the constitution of the urine, so that when secreted in the kidneys and passing through the bladder it no longer contains any insoluble substances of a nature to form precipitates.

9. Carlsbad has also acquired a considerable reputation for its eminently beneficial influence on *gout* and *chronic rheumatism.*

Although the treatment cannot *always* dissolve the deposits of uric acid or the calcareous concretions in and around the joints, still they diminish the frequency, the duration, and the intensity of the attacks; they also alleviate, or often in whole or in part put an end to, the local lesions, to the congestions, the stiffness of the ligaments, and the contractions of the muscles which are the effects of the paroxysms.

It is important for gouty people, after leaving Carlsbad, to continue the use of alkaline waters if they would not rapidly lose the benefits of the thermal treatment, which, in order to insure success, should, if required, be repeated for at least three consecutive years.

10. Clinical experience has proved that the stimulating effect of the hot alkaline springs on the skin and gastro-intestinal membrane, the activity given to the functions of assimilation, enervation, and secretion, have very often removed the beginning of *Bright's disease*, as well as congestion of the kidneys generally. *Albuminuria* at a certain point (when not complicated by any serious organic disorder) has very often been not only relieved, but when the use of the waters is combined with a tonic and strengthening regimen there is good reason to expect even a complete recovery.

11. There is another disease, the result of a general neurosis, affecting all the nerves which govern the secretions—a neurosis resulting in an increased production of sugar in the system, and modifying the

chemical composition of the fluids in the animal economy, not less important by its gravity than by its increasing frequency, which requires as a remedy a sufficient quantity of alkali—that is, *Diabetes*. Scrupulous observation, as well as experience in numerous cases, has shown that these waters are particularly efficacious in diabetes and its consequences.

The excessive secretion from the kidneys charged with sugar, excessive appetite and thirst, dryness of the skin, emaciation, loss of the hair and teeth, eczema, boils and carbuncles, great mental depression—all of these complaints become less distressing during the residence at Carlsbad, provided the waters are taken in time and the prescribed antidiabetic regimen strictly adhered to.

All, in fact, obtain here in a short time very great relief, and many of the above-mentioned symptoms disappear entirely.

The sugar in the urine disappears gradually and in time completely. The thirst is assuaged, the general strength is restored, calm succeeds to uneasiness, and sleep to wakefulness. The relief obtained may be a result of the tonic action and of the stimulating properties which almost all mineral waters exercise on the skin, on the secretions, and on the functions in general. Or, again, the real cause of the benefit derived by diabetic patients may be in consequence of the chemical composition and alkaline properties of the water, which acts as a very useful adjuvant, or specific and sovereign remedy in cases of diabetes.

12. The Carlsbad waters are of the greatest use in the treatment of *Hæmorrhöids* (piles), a very distressing condition, which arise from abdominal disorders. Patients with the most alarming symptons, such as giddiness, congestions, hæmorrhage, asthma, itching and burning of the skin, are very often freed from the complaint, as the blind piles burst and a hæmorrhöidal flux results from the use of the waters.

13. Also general *obesity* as well as *local deposition of fat* in the intestinal organs of the chest and abdomen and their consecutive symptoms, as asthma, congestion, different disorders of the digestion, weakness, &c., undergo a remarkable improvement by a prolonged residence at Carlsbad.

14. Also *Prosopalgia* (Fothergill's pain, Tic-douloureux) as well as *Migraine*, which are not infrequently a consequence of plethora abdominalis, are very often greatly benefited here.

15. *Diseases of the sexual system*, such as Metritis chronica, swelling of the ostium uterinale, menstrual derangements, swelling of the ovaries, sterility—all these female complaints (especially if they arise in consequence of plethora abdominalis, even if the state is chronic and the character is atonic), derive much advantage and improvement from a course of these waters. The efficacy of the Carlsbad water in the treatment of these diseases is often greatly assisted at the same time by the use of the peat baths and the local application of peat poultices.

Hypochondriasis, *Hysteria*, and *Melancholia*, which have their origin in disorders of the abdominal organs; symptoms of stagnation of blood in the liver, in the spleen, in the pancreas, and in the uterus; *symptoms of suppressed and irregular catamenia*—in all these cases the use of Carlsbad water has a powerful effect.

The change of climate, picturesque scenery, and pleasant companions also largely contribute to the restoration of the health of invalids.

VI.

PERIOD AT WHICH THE EFFECT OF THE WATERS MANIFESTS ITSELF.

THERE is no fallacy more widely spread and none less based on reason and experience than the expectation of immediate or even rapid results from the treatment by natural mineral waters of such diseases as are amenable to this efficacious and permanently beneficent therapeutic agency when properly applied. Patients are frequently disappointed and often lose hope if urgent symptoms are not quickly relieved or do not yield to treatment as they may be expected to do in acute disease, in which remedies are usually heroic in their application, and when successful more or less quickly manifest their effects.

It must not be forgotten that most, if not all, of those affections for which hydrotherapeutics are adapted are not only chronic in character, but are also usually of long standing. In numberless cases they are due to hereditary causes or to the habits of a lifetime, and produce results, functional and organic, which it would not be safe to attempt to change suddenly, even if it were practicable to attain this result. What is slow of growth and becomes ingrafted in the constitution can only gradually be changed surely and safely.

"Chi va piano va sano, e chi va sano va lontano," says a good Italian proverb. In many cases of some affections, such as gout in several of its protean forms, scrofulous disease, and not a few acquired affections, the immediate result of a course of mineral water treatment is not only not manifest at all until some time afterwards, but needs renewal for several seasons before a permanent cure can be effected. Hence no patient should lose heart or abandon hope, even if there is no magician's wand in the hands of his physician to perform miracles in the relief of his sufferings.

PRINTED BY BALLANTYNE, HANSON AND CO.
EDINBURGH AND LONDON.

CARLSBAD.

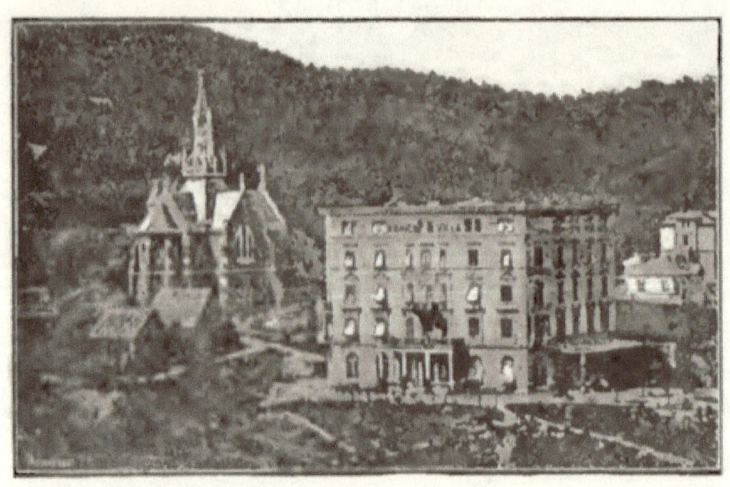

PENSION KÖNIGS-VILLA,
WESTEND-GARDEN.

BEST SITUATION ON THE SCHLOSSBERG,
With Splendid Views of the Neighbouring Mountains.

Very Pleasant Rooms, Large Dining Hall, Drawing and Reading Rooms, with English and American Newspapers.

Meals at fixed prices, à la carte, and at any time of the day.

ENGLISH ATTENDANCE.

W. FASOLT, Proprietor.

Carlsbad. | **HOTEL DE HANOVRE.** | Carlsbad.

FIRST CLASS HOTEL,

Situated in the Centre of the Town, opposite the Post and Telegraph Offices, near the Springs, Curhaus, and Promenades, offering every comfort to Visitors who come for the benefit of the Waters.

Well-Furnished Apartments for Families, with good Attendance.

Cuisine and strictly moderate charges.

C. H. ZORKENDORFER, Proprietor.

LOW'S STANDARD NOVELS.

In small post 8vo, uniform, red cloth, bevelled boards.
Price 6s. each, unless where otherwise stated.

By WILLIAM BLACK.

Three Feathers.	In Silk Attire.
A Daughter of Heth (19th Edition).	Lady Silverdale's Sweetheart.
Kilmeny.	Sunrise.

By R. D. BLACKMORE.

Lorna Doone (25th Edition). Also an Illustrated Edition, 31s. 6d. and 35s.	Cripps the Carrier.
	Erema; or, My Father's Sin.
Alice Lorraine.	Mary Anerley.
Cradock Nowell.	Christowell: a Dartmoor Tale.
Clara Vaughan.	Tommy Upmore.

By THOMAS HARDY.

The Trumpet-Major.	Two on a Tower.
Far from the Madding Crowd.	A Pair of Blue Eyes.
The Hand of Ethelberta.	The Return of the Native.
A Laodicean.	

By GEORGE MacDONALD.

Mary Marston.	Stephen Archer.
Guild Court.	Weighed and Wanting.
The Vicar's Daughter.	Orts.
Adela Cathcart.	

Low's Standard Novels—*continued.*

By Mrs. J. H. RIDDELL.

Daisies and Buttercups: a Novel of the Upper Thames.
The Senior Partner.
Alaric Spenceley.
A Struggle for Fame.

By Mrs. CASHEL HOEY.

A Golden Sorrow (New Edition). | Out of Court.

By W. CLARK RUSSELL.

Wreck of the "Grosvenor."
John Holdsworth (Chief Mate).
A Sailor's Sweetheart.
The "Lady Maud."
Little Loo: A Tale of South Sea.
A Sea Queen.
Jack's Courtship.
My Watch Below.

By Mrs. BEECHER STOWE.

My Wife and I.
Old Town Folk.
We and Our Neighbours.
Poganuc People.

By Mrs. B. M. CROKER.

Some One Else.

By JEAN INGELOW.

Don John. | Sarah de Beranger.

By Mrs. MACQUOID.

Elinor Dryden. | Diane.

By Miss COLERIDGE.

An English Squire.

By the Rev. E. GILLIAT, M.A.

A Story of the Dragonades.

By JOSEPH HATTON.

Three Recruits, and the Girls they Left Behind Them.

By C. F. WOOLSON.

Anne. | For the Major. Price 5s.

By LEWIS WALLACE.

Ben Hur: a Tale of the Christ.

SAMPSON LOW, MARSTON & CO.'S
NEW BOOKS OF TRAVEL.

Now ready, crown 8vo, Illustrated, cloth extra, 7s. 6d.
MOUNTAIN ASCENTS IN WESTMORELAND AND CUMBERLAND.

By JOHN BARROW, F.R.S., Member of the Alpine Club, Lieut.-Col. late 18th Middlesex Rifle Regt. (5th Vol. Batt. Rifle Brigade), Author of "Expeditions on the Glaciers," &c.

THROUGH THE KALAHARI DESERT:

A Narrative of a Journey with Gun, Camera, and Note-Book to Lake N'Gami and Back.

By G. A. FARINI. With Forty-four Illustrations (mostly from Photographs), Diagram, and Map. Demy 8vo, cloth extra, 21s.

THREE THOUSAND MILES THROUGH BRAZIL.

By JAMES W. WELLS. With over Eighty Illustrations. Two Vols. demy 8vo, price 28s.

One Vol. demy 8vo, cloth extra, with numerous Illustrations and Coloured Map. 18s.
NORTH BORNEO.

Explorations and Adventures on the Equator.

By the late FRANK HATTON, Fellow of the Chemical Society and Associate of the Institute of Chemistry of London; Member of the Chemical Society of Berlin, and of the Straits Settlements Branch of the Asiatic Society; and Scientific Explorer in the Service of the British North Borneo Company and Government of Sabah. With Preface by Sir WALTER MEDHURST, and Biographical Sketch by JOSEPH HATTON.

"This book, on a superficially known country, destined probably to rise into brilliant prosperity under British guidance, is sure to be deservedly popular."—*Daily Telegraph.*
"A monument to a bright and promising career."—*Graphic.*

NEW BOOKS OF TRAVEL—*continued*.

Third and Cheaper Edition, crown 8vo, limp cloth, 3s. 6d.
40,000 MILES OVER LAND AND WATER.
The Journal of a Tour through the British Empire and America. By Mrs. HOWARD VINCENT. With numerous Illustrations and a Map of Route.

"Very bright, interesting."—*Morning Post*.
"Deserves and will receive an extended popularity."—*Daily Telegraph*.
"Most charming."—*Vanity Fair*.

EL MAGHREB:
12,000 Miles' Ride through Morocco.
By HUGH E. M. STUTFIELD. With Map. Crown 8vo, cloth, 8s. 6d.

EIGHT MONTHS ON THE GRAN CHACO OF THE ARGENTINE REPUBLIC.
By GIOVANNI PELLESCHI. Crown 8vo, cloth extra, 8s. 6d.

"It is a complete record of life in this little-known forest land, with notes of the scenery and natural productions, of the natives and their customs (with a good deal of philology and racial speculation), and some striking political scenes."—*The Graphic*.
"A pleasant volume well packed with information."—*St. James' Gazette*.

Popular Works of Travel and Adventure.

The Great Lone Land. By Col. W. F. BUTLER, C.B. Illustrated. Cr. 8vo, 7s. 6d.

The Wild North Land. By Col. W. F. BUTLER, C.B. Illustrated. Cr. 8vo, 7s. 6d.

How I Found Livingstone. By H. M. STANLEY. Illustrations and Maps. Cr. 8vo, 7s. 6d.

Through the Dark Continent. By H. M. STANLEY. Numerous Illustrations. Crown 8vo, 12s. 6d.

The Threshold of the Unknown Region. By C. R. MARKHAM. Illustrated. 10s. 6d.

Cruise of the Challenger. By W. J. J. SPRY, R.N. Illustrated. 7s. 6d.

Burnaby's "On Horseback through Asia Minor." With Map. 10s. 6d.

Schweinfurth's "Heart of Africa." Illustrated. Two Vols. 15s.

Marshall's "Through America." Illustrated. 7s. 6d.

LONDON: SAMPSON LOW, MARSTON, SEARLE, & RIVINGTON, CROWN BUILDINGS, 188 FLEET STREET, E.C.

www.ingramcontent.com/pod-product-compliance
Lightning Source LLC
Chambersburg PA
CBHW022011220426
43663CB00007B/1037